Medical Virology

The Practical Approach Series

SERIES EDITORS

D. RICKWOOD
Department of Biology, University of Essex
Wivenhoe Park, Colchester, Essex CO4 3SQ, UK

B. D. HAMES
Department of Biochemistry and Molecular Biology
University of Leeds, Leeds LS2 9JT, UK

Affinity Chromatography
Anaerobic Microbiology
Animal Cell Culture
  (2nd Edition)
Animal Virus Pathogenesis
Antibodies I and II
Basic Cell Culture
Behavioural Neuroscience
Biochemical Toxicology
Biological Data Analysis
Biological Membranes
Biomechanics—Materials
Biomechanics—Structures and
  Systems
Biosensors
Carbohydrate Analysis
  (2nd Edition)
Cell–Cell Interactions
The Cell Cycle
Cell Growth and Division
Cellular Calcium
Cellular Interactions in
  Development
Cellular Neurobiology

Centrifugation (2nd Edition)
Clinical Immunology
Computers in Microbiology
Crystallization of Nucleic Acids
  and Proteins
Cytokines
The Cytoskeleton
Diagnostic Molecular Pathology
  I and II
Directed Mutagenesis
DNA Cloning I, II, and III
Drosophila
Electron Microscopy in Biology
Electron Microscopy in
  Molecular Biology
Electrophysiology
Enzyme Assays
Essential Developmental
  Biology
Essential Molecular Biology I
  and II
Experimental Neuroanatomy
Extracellular Matrix
Fermentation

Medical Virology

A Practical Approach

Edited by

U. DESSELBERGER

Clinical Microbiology and Public Health Laboratory,
Addenbrooke's Hospital, Cambridge, UK

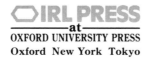

OXFORD UNIVERSITY PRESS
Oxford New York Tokyo

Oxford University Press, Walton Street, Oxford OX2 6DP
Oxford   New York
Athens   Auckland   Bangkok   Bombay
Calcutta   Cape Town   Dar es Salaam   Delhi
Florence   Hong Kong   Istanbul   Karachi
Kuala Lumpur   Madras   Madrid   Melbourne
Mexico City   Nairobi   Paris   Singapore
Taipei   Tokyo   Toronto
and associated companies in
Berlin   Ibadan

Oxford is a trade mark of Oxford University Press

Published in the United States
by Oxford University Press Inc., New York

A catalogue record for this book is available from the British Library

Library of Congress Cataloging-in-Publication Data
Medical virology : a practical approach / edited by U. Desselberger.
p.   cm. — (The practical approach series ; 147)
Includes bibliographical references and index.
1. Medical virology—Laboratory manuals.   I. Desselberger, U.
II. Series
[DNLM: 1. Virus Diseases—diagnosis.   2. Virus Diseases—therapy.
3. Viruses. WC 500 M489 1995]
QR201.V55M43   1995   616'.0194—dc20   95–29781
ISBN 0 19 963330 4 (Hbk)
ISBN 0 19 963329 0 (Pbk)

Typeset by Footnote Graphics, Warminster, Wilts
Printed in Great Britain by Information Press Ltd, Eynsham, Oxon.

Preface

Like other biomedical sciences, medical virology has undergone a revolution of diagnostic and scientific approaches through the advent of molecular biological techniques. The topics collected in this volume reflect this.

C. R. Madeley (Chapter 1) has given a broad description of many 'classical' techniques in viral diagnosis. J. J. Gray and T. G. Wreghitt (Chapter 2) have provided an overview of versions of immunoassays in use. J. Clewley (Chapter 3) has dealt with nucleic acid detection by extraction and hybridization. Applications of blotting procedures for viral proteins are described by S. E. Adams and N. R. Burns in Chapter 4. P. Simmonds has summarized his experience with the polymerase chain reaction for the purpose of viral diagnosis (Chapter 5). D. Kinchington, H. Kangro, and D. J. Jeffries (Chapter 6) discuss basic techniques for the evaluation of antiviral compounds. U. Desselberger (Chapter 7) has described the application of various molecular techniques to aspects of the epidemiology of virus infections, and A. J. Leigh Brown (Chapter 8) has provided a discussion of basic principles of and practical approaches to the analysis of viral evolution.

Although there is some overlap with other issues of the *Practical Approach* series, in particular M. B. A. Oldstone's *Molecular Pathogenesis* and A. Davison's and R. M. Elliott's *Molecular Virology*, the authors of this volume hope to elicit the interest of medical virologists, microbiologists, and physicians with this collection of procedures and the results emanating from them.

Development in the science of virology is rapid, and more refined techniques continuously enter the field of medical applications. It is one of the challenges of medical virology of today to develop and maintain an appropriate mixture of classical and molecular techniques for viral analysis, and if this volume can contribute to the discussion of such issues, it fulfils its purpose.

Cambridge   U.D.
January 1994

Contents

3. Nucleic acid detection 57

Jonathan P. Clewley

4. Blotting of viral proteins 83

Sally E. Adams and Nigel R. Burns

5. Polymerase chain reaction   107

P. Simmonds

List of contributors

SALLY E. ADAMS
British Biotech plc, Watlington Road, Oxford OX4 5LY, UK.

NIGEL R. BURNS
British Biotech plc, Watlington Road, Oxford OX4 5LY, UK.

JONATHAN P. CLEWLEY
Virus Reference Division, Central Public Health Laboratory, 61 Colindale Avenue, London NW9 5HT, UK.

U. DESSELBERGER
Clinical Microbiology and Public Health Laboratory, Level 6, Addenbrooke's Hospital, Hills Road, Cambridge CB2 2QW, UK.

J. J. GRAY
Clinical Microbiology and Public Health Laboratory, Level 6, Addenbrooke's Hospital, Hills Road, Cambridge CB2 2QW, UK.

DONALD J. JEFFRIES
Department of Virology, St Bartholomew's Hospital, 51–53 Bartholomew Close, West Smithfield, London EC1A 7BE, UK.

HILLAR KANGRO
Department of Virology, Serum Institute, Artillerivej 5, 2300 Copenhagen, Denmark.

DEREK KINCHINGTON
Department of Virology, St Bartholomew's Hospital, 51–53 Bartholomew Close, West Smithfield, London EC1A 7BE, UK.

ANDREW J. LEIGH BROWN
Centre for HIV Research, Division of Biological Sciences, University of Edinburgh, West Mains Road, Edinburgh EH9 3JN, UK.

C. R. MADELEY
Department of Virology, Royal Victoria Infirmary and Division of Virology, University of Newcastle, Newcastle-upon-Tyne NE1 4LP, UK.

P. SIMMONDS
Department of Medical Microbiology, University of Edinburgh, Teviot Place, Edinburgh EH8 9AG, UK.

T. G. WREGHITT
Clinical Microbiology and Public Health Laboratory, Level 6, Addenbrooke's Hospital, Hills Road, Cambridge CB2 2QW, UK.

Abbreviations

ACV	acyclovir
APS	ammonium persulphate
BAL	bronchoalveolar lavage
BPL	β-propiolactone
BSA	bovine serum albumin
CD_{50}	cytotoxic dose 50 per cent
CFT	complement fixation test
CMC	carboxymethyl cellulose
CMV	cytomegalovirus
CPE	cytopathic effect
CSF	cerebrospinal fluid
DAB	diaminobenzidine
DEAFF	detection of early antigen by fluorescent foci
DEPC	diethyl pyrocarbonate
DMSO	dimethylsulphoxide
ds	double stranded
DTT	dithiothreitol
EBV	Epstein–Barr virus
EDTA	ethylenediamine tetraacetic acid
EIA	enzyme immuno-assay
ELISA	enzyme-linked immonosorbent assay
EM	electron microscopy
FBS	fetal bovine serum
GuSCN	guanidinium thiocyanate
HA	haemagglutinin
HBV	hepatitis B virus
HCV	hepatitis C virus
HIV	human immunodeficiency virus
HPV	human papillomavirus
HSV	herpes simplex virus
HTLV	human T-cell leukaemia virus
IC_{50}	inhibitory concentration 50 percent
IEM	immuno-electron microscopy
IF	immunofluorescence
mAb	monoclonal antibody
NBT	nitroblue tetrazolium
NPA	nasopharyngeal aspirate
NRS	normal rabbit serum
PAGE	polyacrylamide gel electrophoresis

PBMC	peripheral blood mononuclear cells
PBS	phosphate-buffered saline
PCR	polymerase chain reaction
PHLS	Public Health Laboratory Service
PMSF	phenylmethylsulphonyl fluoride
PVDF	polyvinyldifluoride
RBCs	red blood cells
RI	refractive index
RIA	radioimmunoassay
RSV	respiratory syncytial virus
SD	standard deviation
SI	selectivity index
SDS	sodium dodecyl sulphate
ss	single stranded
TCA	trichloroacetic acid
$TCID_{50}$	tissue culture infective dose 50 per cent
TEMED	N,N,N',N'-tetramethylethylene diamine
TK	thymidine kinase
VRC	vanadyl-ribonucleoside complex
VTM	virus transport medium
WHO	World Health Organization

Traditional techniques of viral diagnosis

C. R. MADELEY

1. Rationale of virus diagnosis

There are three principal reasons for diagnosing infections by viruses:

(a) where treatment or management (isolation, termination of pregnancy, etc.) depends on the diagnosis;

(b) where confirmation of the cause provides confidence in handling the patient, avoiding the use of antibiotics or further investigation and, in some cases, allowing earlier discharge from hospital;

(c) to acquire epidemiological data.

In the first two, speed in making the diagnosis is clearly important while in the third, completeness is more important. In all, accuracy is essential. Although up to 5% of errors may be statistically insignificant in epidemiological terms, such a level is not acceptable scientifically, and most laboratories achieve better results than this. However, diagnostic virology until now has been largely a do-it-yourself trade with the staff of laboratories developing tests to answer local questions and to follow individual interests. The advent of monoclonal antibodies (mAbs) has opened the way to the production of reliable commercial kits and the possibility of more standardization in laboratory practice.

If treatment and management of the patient based on specific diagnosis are to be realistic aims, the results must be available as soon as possible. In the last ten to fifteen years new techniques of rapid diagnosis have been developed and evaluated. While not all infections can yet be diagnosed within one working day, this is the ideal and is now achievable for many viruses although the techniques have not yet been adopted universally. In the sections which follow, emphasis and priority will be given to rapid diagnosis. As new drugs for treating virus infections become available, rapid techniques will become even more essential. There is no virtue in knowing which drug is appropriate when it is too late to use it.

Even if no drug is, or is likely to become, available, the value of a specific diagnosis in avoiding further unnecessary, and often expensive, diagnostic tests should not be underestimated. If the additional reassurance of certainty, in contrast to the guess that 'It's probably a virus', is added there is a powerful argument for identifying the culprit virus even in the cost-conscious 1990s.

For rapid diagnosis, serology has a limited role. The first serum antibody to appear after primary infection is of the IgM class. This is reliably detectable about 1 week after onset when, in most infections, virus replication is over. However, there is value in looking for antibody for the following reasons:

(a) The onset of illness due to the antibiotic-sensitive organisms *Coxiella burnetii*, chlamydiae (*Chlamydia psittaci*, *C. trachomatis*, and *C. pneumoniae*), and *Mycoplasma pneumoniae* is insidious. These organisms are difficult and/or dangerous to isolate, and antibody levels have often risen by the time diagnosis is sought. Traditionally, diagnosis of infections caused by them is done by virus laboratories, and this situation appears unlikely to change.

(b) There is an existing need for assessing immunity to a variety of viruses, e.g. rubellavirus and poliovirus. This is being steadily extended by new demands. Previous infections by cytomegalovirus (CMV) and varicella-zoster must be assessed before transplant operations, and levels of antibody to hepatitis B virus must be assessed after immunization. Antibody tests are also central to investigating infections with human immunodeficiency virus.

(c) Antibody tests are a useful back-up to tests for viruses or viral components. For various reasons specimens for the latter may be taken inappropriately or too late.

(d) The appearance (or persistence) of IgM class antibody is evidence for recent (or continuing) virus activity.

These arguments point to the need for a comprehensive diagnostic service covering all possibilities, but few laboratories provide this. They cover local regular needs and refer other specimens to specialist or reference laboratories. There is no advantage in providing tests which are used infrequently; most tests work best when in regular and frequent use. The laboratory should also take the lead in developing the service, based on discussions with the clinicians who will benefit from any changes.

The sections that follow outline the traditional techniques used in diagnostic laboratories with their advantages and disadvantages.

2. Detection of virus or viral antigen

This is the province of rapid diagnosis supported and supplemented by cell culture. In many cases a useful diagnosis can be provided within one working day. Cell culture, which can take weeks to show detectable infection, is regarded as the gold standard by which other techniques are measured. Although not all viruses grow in cell culture, cell culture is necessary to assess virus viability, and indicates both active infection and its potential for transmission. It provides virus for further investigation and the seed material for developing new tests and controlling old ones for quality.

Some methods combine cell culture with, for example, immunofluorescence and therefore seem more elaborate. They are necessary where suitable specimens for rapid diagnosis are unobtainable and/or the virus grows too slowly.

In the sections on techniques which follow, the techniques are discussed roughly in descending order of speed but, as will be seen, there is considerable overlap, and absolute speed will be compromised by the need to process specimens in batches for convenience and economy.

2.1 Electron microscopy

One characteristic virus particle seen in the microscope makes the diagnosis: the speed of diagnosis by this method can be matched only by latex agglutination tests, and the certainty of diagnosis (in identifying the morphology of the virus) can be matched by none. However, there are limitations which must be recognized (see below) beginning with that imposed by insufficient virus being present in the specimen. This limits the contexts in which electron microscopy (EM) can be used; these limitations are listed in *Table 1*.

Not all these contexts are of equal importance. With the elimination of smallpox, the vesicular rashes requiring diagnosis are usually atypical ones in immunocompromised patients. As seen in *Table 2*, most of the use of EM diagnosis (based on 1989 figures) in the UK Public Health Laboratory Service (PHLS) has been to examine faecal extracts from patients with diarrhoea. Whether this predominance will change with time depends on the availability, reliability, and cost of other techniques. The major cost of EM is providing the facility in the first place—using it is comparatively cheap. There are advantages and disadvantages of EM which should be recognized; they are outlined in *Table 3*. For two reasons, the advantages outweigh the disadvantages: firstly, speed, and secondly, the absence of satisfactory alternatives to detect the variety and multiplicity of viruses in diarrhoeal faeces.

In the context of routine diagnosis, EM means the use of negative contrast —mixing an electron-dense, non-crystalline salt solution with an aqueous suspension of the specimen from the patient, allowing time for reaction, applying the mixture to a microscope grid, removing the surplus, and examining the grid for virus particles after it has dried. Thin section methods are too slow to be useful for rapid diagnosis and the appearance of the particles is less characteristic. The negative stain used routinely by most microscopists is potassium phosphotungstate, usually at a nominal concentration of 3% and at neutral pH. These conditions provide good contrast and help virus particles to stand out against background debris. However, other stains are useful in

Table 1. Contexts in which electron in microscopy can be used in virus diagnosis

1. Where handling of the patient or treatment depends on immediate diagnosis:
   (a) for herpetic vesicular rashes—caused by herpes simplex and varicella-zoster viruses
   (b) for other vesicular rashes due to, for instance, poxviruses such as monkeypox, whitepox variants, and cowpox
2. Viruses which grow with difficulty or not at all
   (a) Viruses which are associated with diarrhoea, singly or as multiple infections
       i. in endemic diarrhoea, particularly in childhood and old age
       ii. in epidemic diarrhoea at all ages
   (b) Viruses in skin lesions
       i. warts, common or genital
       ii. molluscum contagiosum
       iii. orf/pseudocowpox
   (c) viruses in serum
       i. parvovirus B19
       ii. hepatitis B virus [a]
3. Viruses in urine
   (a) CMV in congenitally infected infants [b]
   (b) BK virus in immunosuppressed patients [c]
4. Confirmation of virus in cell culture
   (a) non-neutralizable 'virus' [d]
   (b) atypical CPE [d]
   (c) distinguishing mixed infections
5. Other contexts
   (a) viral meningitis (in cerebrospinal fluid) [a]
   (b) respiratory viruses in throat washings [a]
   (c) eye infections due to viruses [e]
   (d) any other contexts in which the operator can use his/her ingenuity to obtain virus from the patient in sufficient concentration.

[a] Demonstrated to be possible but rarely used.
[b] Virus rarely, if ever, reaches detectable levels in the urine of older immunosuppressed patients although undoubtedly present in a proportion.
[c] Comparatively frequent although significance is not known.
[d] May be due to toxicity of the specimen or a passenger virus from the species of origin—e.g. foamy agent or SV40 in monkey cells.
[e] Shown to be possible but yet to be evaluated.

---

particular circumstances and a choice should be available, both of stains and different pH values. (*Table 4*).

2.1.1 Specimen preparation

The intention is to put as much 'clean' virus, properly stained, on the grid as possible. Some specimens, such as vesicle fluid, require little or no cleaning up and it is necessary only to mix them with an equal volume of stain. The purity of others can be improved by differential centrifugation although some

Table 2. Use of electron microscopy in virus diagnosis (figures from 35 laboratories in the Public Health Laboratory Service in 1989)

Specimen	Numbers examined	% of total
Faeces	52 116	87.9
Cell culture	3 036	5.1
Skin lesions	2 292	3.9
Thin section	744	1.3
Non-viral	384	0.6
Other	732	1.2
Total	59 304	100.0

Table 3. Advantages and disadvantages of electron microscopy

Factor	Comments
Advantages	
Speed	Results may be obtained as early as 10 min after receipt of specimen
Certainty	Only one typical particle confirms the diagnosis
No growth needed	Can be used with viruses which do not grow in cell culture
Mixed infections shown	Common in gut infections
No antiserum needed	No need to decide beforehand which viruses are to be sought
Catch-all technique	Demonstrates all viruses present in sufficient concentration, including 'new' viruses
Disadvantages	
Insensitivity	At least 10^6 particles/ml required
Lack of discrimination	Viruses with similar morphologies cannot be distinguished except with special techniques. Best examples are herpes simplex and varicella-zoster viruses which are totally indistinguishable by EM, though antigenically distinct.
Low throughput	About four specimens/hour; unsuitable generally for large-scale surveys
Extravagance	Experienced, trained operator needed (and in practice)
Expensive	Expensive to buy and maintain but not to use; becomes cheaper the more it is used.

virus is inevitably lost in the pellet discarded after the initial low-speed spin (*c.* 3000 r.p.m. (900 *g*) for 15 min). A subsequent spin at 100 000 *g* for 1 h is considerably more than is necessary to sediment even the smallest viruses but appears to do the particles no harm, and avoids tailoring the centrifuge parameters to the viruses thought likely to occur in the specimen. Because the

Table 4. Negative stains[a]

Stain	pH	Comments
Potassium phosphotungstate (KPT)	3% phosphotungstic acid adjusted to pH 7.0 with 1 M KOH	Best routine stain, good contrast; good contast; will disrupt membranes, including viral envelopes, with time
Ammonium molybdate	7.0	Less contrast than KPT but less disruptive to membranes
Uranyl acetate	3.5	Insoluble at higher pH values; poor contrast but good in revealing structural detail; produces the most elegant pictures
Uranyl formate	3.5	Unstable—has to be prepared fresh; shows the finest detail but tedious to use; poor contrast makes it easy to miss virus particles

[a] Other stains such as sodium silicotungstate and methylamine tungstate are also available but have not shown any notable advantage over the above.

high speed pellet can be substantial, particularly from stool extracts, the amount of dilution necessary to be able to achieve a translucent suspension may mean that the high-speed spin is not really a concentration step. Its main value is to allow removal of salt and soluble protein, both of which can obscure either the particles or details on their surface. Our routine technique is outlined in *Protocol 1*.

Protocol 1. Preparation of specimens for electron microscopy

A. *Stool specimens*

1. Take 1–2 g of faecal material in a 1 oz universal.
2. Add 5–10 ml of phosphate-buffered saline.
3. Re-cap firmly and shake briskly by hand until the material is well dispersed. (Glass beads may be added if necessary.)
4. Clarify by centrifugation at 3000 r.p.m. (900 g) for 15 min in bench centrifuge.
5. Remove aliquot of supernatant for culture if required.
6. Transfer further supernatant to ultracentrifuge tube. Top up with distilled water (if necessary).
7. Centrifuge in a swing-out rotor at approximately 100 000 g for 1 h.

8. Pour off supernatant into 1% hypochlorite solution and plug tube with piece of paper tissue or towel while inverted. Allow to drain in this position.

9. When dry, discard tissue or towel into hypochlorite solution.

10. Add one or two drops (equivalent to 25–50 µl) of 0.01% bacitracin (as wetting agent) in distilled water to the pellet and carefully resuspend (avoiding frothing) with a Pasteur pipette. Continue washing up and down until a smooth suspension is obtained.

11. Transfer one drop of suspension to a piece of dental wax[a] measuring about 2 cm × 1 cm. Add a further drop of bacitracin diluent to the wax and dilute suspension as necessary to produce a faintly opalescent density.

12. Mix a small quantity with an equal volume of suitable negative stain[b] and apply a drop of the mixture to a carbon/Formvar-coated 400 mesh copper EM grid.

13. Draw off the surplus mixture with the torn edge of a piece of filter paper.

14. Allow the grid to dry and examine in the microscope.

B. *Urine and serum specimens*

Proceed from step 6 above.

C. *Vesicle fluid in a syringe*

1. Carefully rinse out vesicle fluid with a small amount of bacitracin diluent on to a piece of dental wax (see step 11 above).

2. Mix one drop with an equal volume of negative stain (usually potassium phosphotungstate) and proceed as from step 12 above.

D. *Skin biopsies*

1. Grind in a chilled (−20 °C) mortar with a pestle, with a small amount of sterile sand and distilled water.

2. Transfer slurry to a conical centrifuge tube. Allow to stand and prepare a small amount of the supernatant as from step 11 above.

[a] As a non-wetting clean surface. Wax impregnated filter paper or Parafilm may be used instead.
[b] See *Table 4*.

As an alternative to centrifugation, the aqueous suspension of the specimen (for example, faeces as an approximate 10% preparation) can be mixed with an equal volume of saturated ammonium sulphate. Proteins, including viruses, are precipitated by low speed centrifugation. The precipitate can be resuspended in a minimal quantity of distilled water, mixed with stain, and examined. This may prevent the disruption of some enveloped viruses but is liable to give a dirtier preparation.

Other concentrating devices such as Lyphogel® which absorb water but not particles have also been tried out. In my experience they appear to remove not only water but also virus, and may convert a positive to a negative, so I would not recommend them.

2.1.2 Enhancement

Two fears haunt diagnostic microscopists—firstly, that there is a lot of virus in the specimen but that the concentration is just below the threshold of detection and, secondly, that virus is visible but unrecognized as virus. Both fears may be alleviated (if not totally removed) by the use of antibody. This can be used in at least three ways: in immuno-electron microscopy (IEM), in solid phase IEM (SPIEM), or as a decoration coupled to a label such as colloidal gold (1).

In the IEM procedure, virus and antibody (diluted with serum as appropriate) are mixed, and immune complexes form in which, at antibody excess, it may be difficult to recognize the virus. This technique works best with a potent antiserum and purified virus. In the SPIEM procedure the grid is coated with antibody to make it 'sticky' for virus particles. Careful washing will leave more particles visible on the grid (up to 100 times more than the routine EM control).

Colloidal gold provides a visible marker for the antibody and can identify not only virus particles but also membranes bearing viral antigens. Such materials may be used to label antibody, either attached directly or as labelled anti-globulin, but gold-labelled immunoglobulin has a short shelf-life. Since it, and other antibodies, may label viral antigens on cell debris, it can be difficult to demonstrate that the sera are specific. If mAbs are used, individual antigenic epitopes can be identified. However, the use of such labels is time-consuming and is rarely appropriate to diagnostic work.

The IEM techniques can be used to detect only those viruses and/or serotypes for which antibody is available. By definition they cannot be used on 'new' viruses. This difficulty can be overcome to some extent by the use of normal pooled human gamma-globulin but it may be difficult to be certain that the necessary antibody is present at all, or in high enough concentration. Convalescent sera following infection can be used for investigating outbreaks or further cases. They are of limited value in routine diagnosis and of no value at all at the acute stage.

Antibody can be a valuable enhancer but its use must be subject to critical examination. It is easily mis- or over-interpreted.

2.1.3 Microscope technique

Details of the operation of the microscope are outside the scope of this book. Finding and identifying virus requires considerable EM expertise and familiarity with the appearance of known viruses. It is not a technique in which to dabble; there are too many opportunities to see what is not there or to fail to see what is.

Even for the experienced who can scan a grid faster than the novice, it is impractical to examine the whole of every grid square. The clue to success is to make a good preparation in the first place, and then to pick out promising areas (not too thick, not too thin) and concentrate on them. Some micro-scopists recommend a regular backwards and forwards raster search within these areas. This is more difficult to do than it appears and is necessary only to ensure that the same area is not examined more than once.

Virus is rarely distributed evenly over the grid—there are richer and poorer areas, which are not related to the amount of material present in each. Several separate areas should therefore be examined before pronouncing a specimen negative. Indeed it is important not to decide too quickly: it often pays to have a final look at another part of the grid. Nonetheless, some faecal preparations contain so much virus (up to 10^{12} particles/g) that surely no one could miss it. However, such high titre specimens can distract the operator from noticing the presence of second or even third viruses and can also incline him/her to give up too soon on low titre specimens where the concentration is just above the threshold of detection (about 10^6 particles/ml).

2.1.4 What is a virus?

At one end of the scale, the presence of vast numbers of particles with typical morphology presents no difficulties in diagnosis. Rotaviruses and adenoviruses provide good examples. At the other, if searches reveal only a few particles (as few as one or two) with no distinguishing features, the microscopist may remain undecided, however long he looks. Between these extremes lies a continuum of increasing difficulty. An understanding of virus structure will help the operator to assess the probability of an object being a virus. Some viruses have characteristic features, making it easier, in theory, to identify them. For example, rotaviruses and adenoviruses should be easy to distinguish but a decayed adenovirus can resemble a protein-covered rotavirus. Similarly, the occasional reovirus can be mistaken for a rotavirus.

In the absence of characteristic features scoring particles as definitely virus may be intuitive. In such doubtful circumstances the number of particles present will have a strong influence, certainty increasing with numbers. In all cases, a micrograph of representative particles (or the only one!) should be taken. To do so provides practice, proof (if needed) that the particle was there, a reference library of viral structures, and the opportunity to compare them with other, later examples. It is essential, of course, that the microscope is operated at a constant magnification. Modern microscopes are generally very stable, but this should be checked regularly by calibration with fixed beef liver catalase crystals as a standard. Although the magnification may not vary greatly between calibrations, its absolute value in my experience can differ from the manufacturer's figure by as much as 13%.

These and other aspects of diagnostic electron microscopy are discussed in greater detail in references 2–4.

2.2 Immunofluorescence

This technique was introduced into virology when adequately specific antisera were difficult to prepare and fluorescence microscopes were adaptations of research microscopes using transmitted illumination. The ensuing difficulties made immunofluorescence (IF) a technique only for enthusiasts. The availability of highly specific mAbs, and of epifluorescence and interference filters, has made IF a reliable, rapid, standard technique.

Before discussing IF in detail there are two important considerations: any specimen from a patient must contain infected cells, and each specimen must be examined individually. If no antigen-containing cells are collected from the patient, IF cannot provide a reliable diagnosis, positive or negative. Individual examination makes the technique labour-intensive, and the microscopist must be experienced.

2.2.1 Contexts

In theory any lesion caused by a viral infection may yield material for IF provided infected cells can be obtained, the likely causative viruses are known, and antisera to them are available. In practice this limits the contexts mostly to those viruses listed in *Table 5*. A standard procedure to prepare specimens for IF is given in *Protocol 2*.

Protocol 2. Preparation of material for immunofluorescence

The intention is to put infected cells in adequate density on to a defined area of a microscope slide for staining. These cells must be separated as far as possible from mucus or other irrelevant debris.

A. *Preparation of specimens*

1. *Naso-pharyngeal secretions*

   Collect secretions by suction into a mucus trap. Carefully resuspend the mucoid material in a small volume (up to 5 ml) of 0.01 m PBS, pH 7.2 with a Pasteur pipette.

   (a) Transfer the suspension to a sterile 3 inch × 0.5 inch test tube with a silicone rubber bung, adding about 0.5 ml to virus transport medium (VTM)[a] if required for culture.

   (b) Pipette the suspension up and down briskly with a Pasteur pipette to break up the mucus.

   (c) Centrifuge at 1000 r.p.m (300 *g*) in a bench centrifuge at room temperature for 10 min.

(d) Remove and discard the supernatant. Resuspend the pellet in two or three drops of PBS and check for residual mucus. If necessary, add further PBS and re-centrifuge after brisk pipetting.

(e) Distribute the resuspended cells onto areas on Teflon ®-coated slides.[b] Prepare as many areas ('wells') as possible.

(f) Dry the cell suspensions with a hair-dryer on 'cold' setting.

(g) Fix the dried preparations in cold (4 °C) acetone for 10 min. Allow to dry.

2. *Broncho-alveolar lavage fluid*

(a) Add about 0.5 ml of the fluid to VTM for culture.

(b) Centrifuge the remainder and make preparations as indicated in steps (c)–(g) above. Teflon-coated slides with seven circular 'wells'[c] are suitable for these specimens but duplicate square-well preparations for staining with anti-herpes simplex serum should also be made.

3. *Scraping from skin or other lesions*

(a) Carefully remove scabs or superficial debris.

(b) Scrape infected cells from the developing edge of the lesion with a sterile scalpel blade.

(c) Transfer the cells to a drop of saline placed on a 1 cm square marked on a microscope slide with a diamond.

(d) Add further cells to at least one other square.

(e) Using two mounted needles tease the cells into an even suspension with no lumps.

(f) Allow to dry and fix in cold acetone as in steps (f) and (g) above.

B. *Staining procedure*

1. Indirect technique using unconjugated polyclonal or monoclonal antisera.

(a) Add 15 μl of each antiserum to the appropriate well.

(b) Incubate at 37 °C for 30 min in a moist chamber. Do not allow to dry out.

(c) Gently wash off sera with PBS

(d) Rinse in three changes of PBS, 10 min in each at room temperature.

(e) Add 15 μl of appropriate anti-globulin conjugate to each well.

(f) Incubate at 37 °C for 30 min again in a moist chamber.

(g) Gently wash off the conjugates with PBS.

(h) Repeat step (d).

(i) Give a final rinse in distilled water for 1 min.

(j) Dry carefully with a hair dryer on 'cold' setting.

(k) Examine unmounted under oil-immersion using a non-fluorescing oil.

2. Direct technique using conjugated antisera. These will be monoclonal

Protocol 2. *Continued*

and often be commercially available. If the latter, they will usually have instructions for use which should be followed. If no instructions are available, proceed as follows.

(a) Add 15 µl of the conjugated antibody, usually containing Evans Blue as a counterstain, to each well.

(b) Incubate at 37 °C for 15 min in a moist chamber.

(c) Wash off conjugates with PBS.

(d) Rinse in PBS for 5 min at room temperature.

(e) Give final 1 min rinse in distilled water.

(f) Dry with hair dryer.

(g) Mount under coverslip in fluorescence-enhancing mountant and examine under oil-immersion.

[a] VTM: Hanks' balanced salt solution containing phenol red indicator, 50 units/ml penicillin G, 50 µg/ml streptomycin and 0.3% w/v bovine serum albumin.
[b] Available in UK from C. A. Hendley, cat. no. PH 009/W or PH 010/W.
[c] Available from C. A. Hendley, cat. no. PH 013/W

Table 5. Contexts in which immunofluorescence can be used

System	Viruses sought	Viruses not sought
Respiratory	Influenza A virus	Rhinoviruses[a]
	Influenza B virus	Coronaviruses[b]
	Respiratory syncytial virus	Enteroviruses[a]
	Adenovirus	Mumps virus[c]
	Parainfluenza viruses types 1–4	Rubella virus[d]
	Measles virus	Influenza C virus[b]
	Varicella-zoster virus	Epstein–Barr virus[c]
	Herpes simplex virus	Reoviruses[b]
	Cytomegalovirus	
Skin rashes/lesions	Herpes simplex virus	Wart viruses[e]
	Varicella-zoster virus	*Molluscum contagiosum*[e]
		Orf/pseudocowpox[e]
Central nervous system	Herpes simplex virus	Various[f]
Urine	(Cytomegalovirus)[g]	Adenovirus[b]
		BK virus[e]
Others		
Biopsies ⎫	Various as appropriate	Various
Post-mortem tissues ⎭		

[a] Too many serotypes and no group antigen.
[b] Too rare?
[c] No suitable specimen.
[d] Too fleeting.
[e] Easier by EM.
[f] In UK. In other regions where other causes of encephalitis are prevalent and brain biopsies are taken, other viruses may be sought.
[g] Rarely positive.

Because infections by different viruses may present similarly, it is necessary to test the cells from the specimen with antisera to several viruses, but the number can be limited by the number of cells in the specimen. In practice, experienced staff will select the sera to use in the first instance, depending on the time of year and the viruses known to be circulating in the community. For example, it is unnecessary to test respiratory specimens for influenza A and B viruses throughout the year. It is better to concentrate on these viruses during late autumn and winter, usually after serology (see below) has indicated local activity. Similar seasonal arguments apply to parainfluenza type 3 (in summer) but others such as respiratory syncytial virus (RSV) may be found all year in addition to causing major epidemics in winter. The selection of antisera is discussed more fully in reference 5.

2.2.2 Advantages and disadvantages of immunofluorescence

These are outlined in *Table 6*. Apart from the obvious advantage of speed, allowing one to make a diagnosis well within the working day, other advantages are that it provides a feedback on the quality of the specimen and, in some cases, provides a prognosis. With respiratory specimens, quality is a constant problem.

Table 6. Advantages and disadvantages of immunofluorescence

Advantages	Comments
Rapid	Same-day diagnosis—as little as 1 h in emergency
Adequately sensitive	Best if specimens are taken early in the illness
May still be positive after start of antibody production	At this stage it may no longer be possible to isolate virus
Isolation systems not necessary	However, culture back-up is needed to evaluate IF fully
Provides feedback on the quality of specimen	A constant problem with nasopharyngeal aspirates (see below)
Provides some evidence for progress and prognosis	See text
In frozen sections, can show virus distribution in tissue	

Disadvantages	Comments
Possibility of false positives	Due to reagents being insufficiently specific; this can be avoided by attention to detail
Labour-intensive	Important in the 'respiratory season'
Experienced microscopist needed	
Low throughput	
Commercial reagents expensive	But moderate cost per test.

Taking specimens adequate in quantity and quality is uncomfortable for the patient, and the temptation to be perfunctory is strong and not always resisted, particularly with distressed children and those with low platelet counts.

Reduction in the number and brightness of fluorescing cells in successive specimens can indicate progress; in the case of measles infections in the immunocompromised, the presence of a large number of infected giant cells indicates a poor prognosis.

The advantages of IF are somewhat offset by its labour-intensiveness and the need for an experienced microscopist. The acquisition of experience is helped if the laboratory also uses cell cultures to isolate or grow viruses. Otherwise the same experience can be gained through an attachment to another laboratory.

2.2.3 Specimens: collection, transport and preparation

The specimens suitable for IF are listed in *Table 7*. For the best results they should be collected early in the illness and transported to the laboratory on ice, without freezing, as soon as possible. Respiratory specimens are perishable, becoming unreliable for both IF and isolation if undue delay occurs. Secretions, aspirates, sputum, and bronchoalveolar lavages (BALs) should be transported quickly without addition of virus transport medium (VTM). We have found it useful to use wide-mouthed vacuum transport flasks so that specimens are kept cool in transit.

Cells from a skin lesion should be taken by scraping the base and borders of the lesion using a sterile scalpel blade. They should be added to a small drop of saline placed on two or more squares of a Teflon®-coated slide (see footnote[b] of *Protocol 2*). The knot of cells should be teased out with two mounted needles and spread as widely as possible over the squares. It can

---

Table 7. Specimens for immunofluorescence

System	Specimens
Respiratory	Nasopharyngeal aspirate (secretions)[a]
	Sputum[b]
	Tracheal aspirate
	Bronchoalveolar lavage[c]
	Transbronchial biopsy[d]
	Open lung biopsy
	Post-mortem lung
Skin	Lesion scraping
Biopsy	Piece(s) of tissue in virus transport medium

[a] Should be complemented by nose and throat swabs in VTM for virus isolation.
[b] Better after physiotherapy for sputum induction.
[c] The lavage fluids should be pooled before an aliquot is taken for virology as the earlier and later washes do not have the same composition.
[d] Not usually a good source of virus-infected cells.

---

then be allowed to dry and sent unfixed to the laboratory without delay but with some protection over the smear.

Once in the laboratory, respiratory specimens for IF, in particular, are prepared in a negative pressure cabinet (Class I or II). Further manipulations of any specimens found to contain influenza A viruses should then be done in a similar cabinet.

The aim in preparation is to extract infected respiratory cells from other (mostly squamous) cells and mucus, neither of which contribute to the diagnosis. With NPAs, the mucoid specimen is suspended in a small amount (*c.* 5 ml) of PBS, briskly pipetted to break up the mucus, and centrifuged in a bench centrifuge to sediment the cells. The cells are then resuspended in a small amount of PBS, and checked for the presence of remaining mucus (a drop should no longer be 'sticky'), and a drop of the cell suspension placed in as many wells on Teflon-coated microscope slides as possible. A number of wells are needed for testing with the appropriate antisera, allowing for re-peats as necessary. Any spare slides are kept for testing new reagents which must be tried on genuine specimens under routine testing conditions.

The preparations are dried, fixed in cold acetone, and then 'stained' with appropriate antisera. Spare slides are stored at or below −40°C until required.

2.2.4 Antisera

The standard of IF depends on the quality of the antisera used. At first, individual laboratories made their own, usually in rabbits. Virus, crude or purified, was used to immunize one or more animals by protocols which varied widely. 'Good' antisera were something of an accident but contained many unwanted antibodies which had to be removed by adsorption before the serum could be used. Comprehensive adsorption was time-consuming and left a relatively small amount of high titre, 'clean' antiserum. This process had to be repeated for each virus which the laboratory wished to detect. These sera were then used in an indirect IF test with a conjugated anti-globulin. Provided all the antisera were made in one species, only one anti-globulin conjugate was required although this, too, had to be cleaned up by adsorption. Differ-ences in quality of polyclonal antisera made IF a technique which was initially practised by only a few laboratories.

The advent of mAbs has changed the situation profoundly. High titre, highly specific antisera can now be reliably produced in commercial quanti-ties. The main production problems are selecting suitable clones, establishing their credentials for use on clinical specimens, and preparing enough of the preferred mixture to satisfy demand. A mixture of mAbs can offset their narrow specificity; the antigenic epitope recognized by a single mAb is rarely present equally in all clinical specimens.

An increasing number of diagnostic kits is now on the market all based on mAbs. Among them are pooled mAbs for use in IF. Given the reproducible quality of the product, the possibility of unlimited production and the need for an off-the-shelf reagent, these have also been conjugated by the manu-facturers, reversing the trend from indirect IF to direct. Consequently, labor-atories which made little use of IF in the past are now using it regularly.

Kits using mAbs in IF tests are available for RSV, influenza A & B viruses, adenovirus, and herpes simplex viruses (types I and II separately). It has not been easy to make discriminatory mAbs against the different parainfluenza virus types, and the World Health Organization (WHO), producing a kit for use in Third World countries, eventually settled for a single parainfluenza reagent which detected all four types. Infections with measles and varicella-zoster viruses do not usually require laboratory confirmation. However, measles is a major problem in Africa, for example, and an antibody to the virus may be added later to the WHO kit. The need for CMV diagnosis in the immunocompromised (patients with transplants, AIDS, etc.) by early antigen detection (see below) has been met by mAbs to the immediate early antigen.

In my laboratory, we still use a full range of polyclonal antibodies where sensitivity is important and use mAbs in the first instance for speed. The RSV and influenza A and B virus mAbs are used as the first line when these viruses are 'in season' and on specimens arriving late in the day but for routine wide coverage the polyclonal sera retain their position.

Laboratories have to be cost-conscious and the use of *all* reagents on *all* specimens does not make economic sense. How to select which sera to use on an individual specimen depends on experience, knowledge of local epi-demiology and seasonality, and on being able to interpret request forms. This aspect of IF has been treated extensively by McGuckin and Taylor (5).

2.2.5 Enhancement of immunofluoresence

Immunofluorescence can be enhanced using counterstains, fluorescing moun-tants, and anti-complement assays. Counterstains are useful in helping to provide a uniform background against which the fluorescence stands out, but they may also obscure faint positives. In the past naphthalene black was the most frequently used counterstain but this only damps down any background and does not help the focusing problem. Evans Blue, which despite its name stains the background red, is better and is now incorporated in many com-mercial conjugates.

There are several commercial fluorescence-enhancing mountants. Their composition is a trade secret but they enhance *all* fluorescence. In practice their use is confined to monoclonal IF conjugates.

In anti-complement assays, complement and an anti-complement antibody conjugate are added after the antiviral antibody has reacted with the speci-men. Further information is given in reference 6. It provides possibly greater sensitivity, but at the cost of a greater risk of false positives and more work on each specimen. It is more of a research tool and is not used routinely by laboratories with a substantial work load.

2.2.6 Detection of early antigen

Throat swabs and urine, as well as the buffy coat of blood, yield CMV by culture but too slowly to be useful in patient management. The lack of a suitable specimen on which CMV infection could be diagnosed early led to an alternative approach. Early antigens are produced only a few hours after infecting cells in culture, and it is the delay in producing the later antigens which makes complete virus production slow. The DEAFF test (detection of early antigen by fluorescent foci) detects the presence of immediate early CMV antigens in coverslip cultures of human diploid fibroblasts using mAbs to the immediate early antigen. The procedure is summarized in *protocol 3*. In brief, specimens are inoculated by low speed centrifugation on to coverslips, and inocula are washed off after 1 h and replaced with culture medium. After incubation overnight (or, if necessary, for longer) the coverslips are stained with the mAb conjugate and examined under a fluorescence microscope. The preparations are usually easy to interpret with infected cells being readily visible. Although slightly less sensitive than long-term culture (for up to 28 days) the DEAFF test provides an answer quickly and is unlikely to miss a high level of infection. It now seems probable that immunoperoxidase staining may be more sensitive than IF.

Protocol 3. Outline protocol for detection of early antigen by fluorescent foci (DEAFF) [a]

1. Prepare coverslip cultures of suitable cells (usually human embryo lung fibroblasts) in plastic vials.
2. Transfer to maintenance medium and use within 7 days.
3. Remove medium by aspiration with a sterile Pasteur pipette and discard.
4. Add 1 ml specimen (in VTM) to two or three coverslips (see step 9).
5. Centrifuge at 600 g (*c.* 2100 r.p.m. in bench top centrifuge) at room temperature for 1 h.
6. Remove specimen with a Pasteur pipette and discard.
7. Add 1 ml of maintenance medium/vial.
8. Incubate vials in 5% CO_2 in air at 37 °C.
9. At appropriate intervals remove vials for staining:-
   (a) for CMV, one after overnight incubation, one after two nights, and one after 7 days
   (b) for herpes simplex virus, one after overnight incubation and one after two nights
   (c) for varicella-zoster virus, one after two nights and one after 14 days

---

Protocol 3. *Continued*

10. Remove medium from vial and rinse in PBS.

11. Fix cells in 1 ml of 75% acetone in PBS for 10 min in an ice bath.

12. Drain and remove coverslip.

13. Attach by one edge to a clean microscope slide with an instant glass-bonding glue.[b]

14. Place on window-sill to polymerize for 10 min.

15. Stain with mAb to immediate early antigen (CMV or equivalent) using indirect technique (see *Protocol 2*). Use 25 µl of antiserum to ensure that the whole coverslip is covered.

16. Examine under oil-immersion after mounting under a second coverslip with fluorescence-enhancing mountant.

[a] Method refined and developed by Dr C. E. Taylor and Miss R. McGuckin, Department of Virology, Newcastle-upon-Tyne, UK.
[b] e.g. Loctite Glass Bond ®.

The same technique has now been adapted to detect herpes simplex virus (which generally grows much more quickly but is sometimes difficult to diagnose by IF from stomatitis) (8) and varicella-zoster which is also a slowly growing virus.

2.2.7 General comments

It is ironic that IF is at last becoming popular some 20 years after it was pioneered. Though labour-intensive it has great value in giving feedback on the quality of the specimen—something not provided by other methods and of practical importance in running a service. With the coming of commercial and reliable mAb conjugates, particularly for RSV, many laboratories with only a marginal interest in virology are now using it in the UK and elsewhere.

The absence of a full set of mAbs to all the common viruses is a drawback, but will be overcome with time. Of possibly greater concern is that all parainfluenza virus types may be lumped together by a non-discriminatory antibody pool. The viruses differ both in epidemiology and the disease they cause, but these patterns could become blurred in the future if a non-discriminatory test is used, raising the more fundamental question of whether a laboratory should provide a complete diagnosis or only a clinically useful one. To take one example, a virologist would want to know if the virus was an echovirus type 9 but a clinician might be satisfied to know only that there was an enterovirus (type unimportant), or a picornavirus, or even simply that *a* virus was definitely present. Personally, I have no doubt about the need for precise diagnosis, for epidemiological reasons if no other. A more complete analysis of IF can be found in references 5 and 7.

2.3 Immunoassays

These are discussed fully in Chapter 2 and warrant an entry here only to put them in context. They can use antibody to detect antigen in the specimen, or antigen to detect antibody of various classes in serum, saliva, cerebrospinal fluid, or faeces. They are conveniently done in microtitre wells either as complete 96-well plates or as 8- or 12-well strips. The end-point is a colour change in the well which can be read by eye or with a spectrophotometer. The latter may be automated and may be attached to a computer which can relate the raw absorbance figures to those in blank wells and in negative and positive controls and give a calculated print-out indicating whether the corrected value is above or below the cut-off level.

Such assays can often be made to work better to detect antibody than antigen in specimens containing a mixture of antigens of which the viral ones are a minority. For antigen detection they have the advantages of being capable of semi-automation, can produce an 'objective' end-point, and can handle large numbers of specimens.

On the negative side they provide no information on the specimen quality or on prognosis—is a specimen negative because there was no virus or because the specimen was inadequate? They often have a 5% error rate which is not significant in population terms but is for individual patients.

2.4 Cell culture

There was a time when no-one could do any virology without cell culture to grow virus in. Now, with the availability of commercial kits and reagents and a great deal known about hepatitis C, a virus no-one has grown or even seen, the necessity of cell culture as an essential component of a diagnostic laboratory has been questioned. But to those who see the unravelling of virus-induced disease as a challenge, the availability of cell culture allows collection of viruses to develop new tests, modify old ones, and provide an alternative if the kit does not work or does not arrive.

On a more mundane level, cell culture has been long thought to be the gold standard in diagnostic virology. It is not hard to see why. It documents infective virus in the patient and indicates definite virus activity. However, failure to grow virus does not rule out recent infection nor does it mean there is no infective virus is present.

Cell culture is expensive, time-consuming, and subject to vagaries and contamination with bacteria and fungi. Despite all this, or perhaps because of it, the presence of cell culture intended to detect all the common cultivatable viruses is a hallmark of serious laboratories which can attempt to sort out problems and adapt to new situations.

2.4.1 Principles

No known single cell type will allow all viruses to grow. Consequently any virologist who wishes to trap as many viruses as possible must expect to keep a variety of cell types available. To do so is a feat somewhere between being a juggler and a successful market gardener.

Many virologists hope that there is, somewhere, the perfect cell line derived from some common unprotected species which will be susceptible not only to all presently cultivable human viruses but to others, such as rotavirus and hepatitis B-type viruses, which have failed to grow routinely, or other viruses about which we know nothing. This is probably a forlorn hope because it is unlikely that any one cell type will bear all the necessary receptors and provide the conditions internally for every virus.

The choice of cell lines is now very large and, since keeping a wide variety is not usually necessary and would put an impossible burden on laboratory staff, it is necessary to select the more appropriate lines. The types of cell available are discussed below. One general rule (but by no means invariable) is that wild strains of virus often grow more readily in cells from their normal host and that primary cells (see below) are more susceptible than continuous cells.

2.4.2 Types of cell

i. Primary cells

Primary cells come from pieces of, usually, adult tissue, minced and dispersed by trypsin or Versene (EDTA) to yield a suspension of individual cells which are seeded into bottles or tubes to form a monolayer. These may be subcultured later to form a secondary culture but the cells do not divide in culture more than two or three times and the cells cannot be passaged further. Although more sensitive to wild-type viruses they have to be prepared afresh each time, and a supply of suitable organs must be available. Primary monkey kidney cells support the replication of a wide variety of human viruses, and virus laboratories used to keep a supply of monkeys in the animal house. Nephrectomies were done routinely as necessary to provide a supply of kidney cells, but these cells are now available commercially.

Another disadvantage of primary cells, apart from the need to renew them frequently, is the likelihood of their having passenger viruses. This is a particular problem with monkey kidney cells which are likely to contain SV5, SV40, or foamy agent. These viruses interfere surprisingly little with the growth of other viruses but may cause difficulties in identifying the infecting virus.

ii. Continuous cell lines

These originate from malignant tissue. They are immortal in that they can be subcultured indefinitely. They carry no passenger viruses, but some continuous cells have been shown to contain virus genomes (for example, the human HeLa cell line, which originated from a cervical malignancy, is known to carry a papillomavirus genome) but these do not appear to be expressed as complete virus. Contrary to the general rule, some continuous cells are the first choice for isolating viruses; this underlines the need to have a variety of cell types available. The main advantage of continuous cells is that providing them routinely is easier than producing primary cells.

iii. Semi-continuous cells

These are fetal in origin, usually from lung, kidney, or liver, although other tissues such as skin or muscle have also been used. For diagnostic virology, lung cells have been most widely used; kidney cells are susceptible to a different spectrum of viruses but are more difficult to obtain. Unlike primary cells, semi-continuous cells will continue to divide in culture but only for up to approximately 70 generations, confirming that they are neither immortal nor malignant. As they approach this limit they become less susceptible to infection, and their performance becomes less predictable. In practice a limit closer to 40 generations is more realistic, but this still gives a very useful life-span. In particular, they provide susceptible cells for two fastidious and common human viruses, CMV and varicella-zoster virus, neither of which will grow in other cells. Over several generations they can be checked for the presence of passenger viruses (rare), and a clean cell culture can be established. It is a pity that these cells, which have such obvious virtues, are not susceptible to a wider range of viruses. With greater public concern over the use of fetal material generally, the long-term availability of such cells may be doubtful. Where fetal tissues can be obtained, laboratories can continue to prepare their own cell lines but similar cells such as MRC-5 and WI-38 are available commercially.

2.4.3 Which cells to choose?

A glance through specialist catalogues shows a vast choice of cell types and lines, most of which have been developed for particular purposes. While a newcomer to cell culture should be willing to experiment, a visit to several diagnostic laboratories will show more similarities than differences in the cell types used routinely. As with other aspects of diagnostic virology, only those cells necessary for the purposes of the laboratory should be obtained. The gardening analogy is a good one, as it is necessary to pay constant attention to keeping out weeds (contamination), feeding the cultures properly and adequately, and providing a good milieu for growth (sufficiently clean glassware or plastics). It is also prudent to handle all cell types as if they were infectious. Obviously, precautions are taken to avoid inhaling or swallowing malignant (continuous) cells, but such cells are also very capable of colonizing other cell types, so all cultures should be handled with caution. Once two cultures are mixed it is impossible to separate them, and hybrids—difficult to achieve deliberately—form readily when you do not want them to.

Table 8 lists some of the more commonly used cell types, with their major virus susceptibilities. In the view of those virologists who remember when they were readily available, rhesus monkey kidney cells are the best primary/secondary cells. They had few passenger viruses and produced good cell sheets, but were chiefly prized for their susceptibility to respiratory viruses, above all to influenza viruses. Their long-term availability is uncertain.

Other primary cells from primates such as African green monkeys and baboons produce more untidy cell sheets with more passenger viruses and are less susceptible to human viruses, particularly influenza viruses. Nevertheless, they are more freely available and less expensive.

No human primary cell lines are available because no healthy organs are removed routinely which could provide a supply. Human cells are represented by continuous cell lines of which HeLa and Hep2 cells are used most widely. These are of cervical and laryngeal origin, respectively. Caco2 cells (from a colonic carcinoma) are being explored as cells which will grow some of the viruses associated with diarrhoea, but have yet to be adopted widely.

Of the continuous cells from non-human sources, different laboratories have their own preferences. Many use Vero, RK13, and BHK21(C13) cells but use of other monkey cell lines (MA104, LLK-MK2, etc.) and of cell lines from other species (KB and L cells from mice) reflects individual needs and preferences. The list in *Table 8* provides a selection from which a new laboratory might choose.

2.4.4 Organization of a cell culture system

Different laboratories have different approaches and methods, so only a few general thoughts are given here. There is no ideal system.

It is better to provide a separate suite of rooms in which uninfected cell cultures are prepared, and it should be well separated from any infected material. Since the preparation of such cell cultures is repetitive and far from exciting, few technicians will want to do it indefinitely. It is, nonetheless, one of the most important jobs in the virus laboratory, and a rotation of senior staff through this section is appropriate. While deployed in the cell culture section, members of staff of the laboratory should avoid the virus isolation areas. In my laboratory, we also separate the handling of continuous cell lines and primary cells into separate rooms to avoid cross-contamination. Similarly, only one cell type is handled at a time, with careful disinfection of the working surfaces between each.

i. Contamination and its prevention

Prevention of bacterial and fungal contamination is a constant concern. Meticulous technique is demanded to keep contamination under control but it may still occur from time to time. Contamination can be introduced by failures in bench technique or through infected components of the culture media. The latter can be monitored by putting an aliquot of each medium

Table 8. Common cell types used for isolating viruses

Origin of cells	Cell types	Species of origin	Other similar cells	Common viruses grown
Primary	Rhesus monkey kidney	*Macaca mulatta*	—	Orthomyxoviruses, paramyxoviruses, enteroviruses
	Baboon kidney[a]	*Papyo hamadryas*	—	Enteroviruses, Herpes simplex viruses, ortho- and paramyxoviruses
	African green monkey kidney	*Cercopithecus aethiops*	Buffalo green monkey (BGM)	
Semi-continuous	Human embryo lung (diploid fibroblasts)	human	MRC-5, WI-38	Cytomegalovirus, varicella-zoster virus, herpes simplex viruses, rhinoviruses
Continuous	HeLa	Human cervical cancer	Various HeLa derivatives	Enteroviruses, respiratory syncytial virus, adenoviruses
	Hep2	Human epithelioma of larynx	KB, Graham 293	Adenoviruses
	Vero	*Cercopithecus aethiops*	MA104, LLC-MK2, BGM	Measlesvirus
	RK13	Rabbit		Rubellavirus

[a] There is considerable variation between batches of these cells in their sensitivity to ortho- and paramyxoviruses.

used and its components into bacteriological broth kept in a hot room for 10 days. This will grow most contaminants which will have to be aerobic to grow in cell cultures.

Aseptic bench technique should become second nature for everyone working in a virology laboratory. This includes no-touch, flaming the necks of tubes and bottles, keeping bungs out and caps off for as short a time as possible, and generally planning the work properly before starting.

Where work is done in Class II cabinets, flaming should not be necessary. A Bunsen burner will affect the air flow in the cabinet and introduces a significant fire risk. A foot-operated valve to a burner designed for use in the cabinet will reduce both air-flow disturbance and the fire-risk.

ii. Choice between glassware and plasticware

Cuts caused by glass tubes or Pasteur pipettes are the commonest form of injury in virus laboratories. As a result their use is discouraged or forbidden with category 3 and 4 viruses. For work with category 2 viruses, which covers the overwhelming majority of viruses isolated routinely, glass is permitted, and the majority of UK laboratories prefer to use glass, because it can be flamed and re-used.

Commercially available plasticware includes tubes (with or without screw-caps), multiwell plates, and individual Petri dishes. It is supplied pre-sterilized and cannot be re-used. As a result it is expensive and provides a considerable volume of infected waste. Plastic items cannot be flamed, except very briefly. They are light in weight and more easily knocked over or out of position than are similar glass items. It is very difficult to prevent cross-contamination between wells in a multiwell plate once the specimens have been inoculated. Individual Petri dishes, however small, are impractical because they are fiddly to handle and have to be kept in a CO_2 gassed incubator. They are also extravagant of cells and culture media.

For dealing with a large number of specimens for isolation, tube cultures provide the only practical solution. On balance, and despite the small hazard of breakages, glass tubes with silicon rubber bungs form the system of choice. They can be re-used (given a good glass-washing system), their necks can be flamed, and they can be handled easily and quickly in considerable numbers. These arguments, both good and bad, also apply to the glass Pasteur pipettes used to inoculate them and change the media as necessary. Plastic ones are not as convenient and take up significantly more space both before and after use.

2.4.5 Virus isolation

There are two main reasons for growing virus from patients: to provide a net in which all those viruses which will grow can be caught, and to isolate complete infectious virus for further investigation. The former provides some degree of 'catch-all', limited to those viruses to which the cells are susceptible, and provides back-up for other techniques such as immunofluorescence targeted towards particular viruses.

As already mentioned, a variety of cell types will be necessary to cover the gamut of likely viruses. Four further factors also need to be considered: the temperature of incubation, whether to roll the cultures, how frequently to change the medium in the tubes, and when to subculture.

i. Temperature

Generally, wild strains of respiratory viruses, and rhinoviruses in particular, grow better at 33°C than at 37°C, possibly because the nasopharyngeal mucosa is cooled by inspired air. A separate 33°C incubator will be needed to complement the usual 37°C hot room.

ii. Rolling cultures

Cultures incubated at 33°C are found to be more sensitive if they are rolled. A roller drum rotating at about one revolution every 8 min can be put in an incubator, or a custom-made roller incubator can be used. Possibly as a result of the medium rolling continually over the cells and presenting repeated virus–cell contact, this procedures raises the rate of virus isolation.

iii. Changing the medium

Metabolizing cells use up the nutrients in the medium and therefore media have to be replaced regularly. How often the medium is changed is usually a matter of laboratory policy. The more frequently tubes are opened, the greater the opportunity for cross-contamination between specimens and the greater the opportunity for bacteria and fungi to enter. The less frequently the medium is replaced, the poorer the cell quality.

iv. Subculturing

Subculturing into fresh cells may be required because the specimen is toxic or because the cells are deteriorating. Some laboratories subculture routinely, others only if obliged to do so. This, again, is a matter of laboratory policy and experience, but providing fresh cultures adds expense.

How long specimens are kept in culture before discarding them is also a matter of policy for the laboratory. The percentage of positive isolations changes with time, reaching a peak (of about 8–10%; this will vary with factors such as the patient mix, quality and quantity of specimens, time from taking to inoculation, the general 'fitness' of the cells, etc.) about 4–6 days after inoculation with a long but low tail. Viruses such as varicella-zoster virus and CMV are inherently slow-growing and may take up to 4 weeks to show, while others such as herpes simplex viruses can produce visible deterioration overnight from a well-taken specimen.

2.4.6 Recognition of virus growth

Virus growth will damage the host cells and cell cultures will deteriorate as a result. Unfortunately, the toxicity of the specimen and ageing of cells in culture will have similar effects. Some viruses produce characteristic cytopathic effects (CPE), like the 'bunches of grapes' caused by adenoviruses, while others induce little visible alteration. Recognizing CPE in unstained cell sheets growing in test-tubes requires practice but very experienced readers claim to be able to recognize virus families and even genera. It is a skill to learn at the bench, not from books. It is complemented by the use of haemadsorption (to pick up influenza and parainfluenza viruses which even at best produce minimal CPE) and EM (to identify the causes of unusual CPE and/or the effects of more than one virus). Since toxicity can produce effects very like viral CPE, EM can save both time and expense in trying to identify or exclude a virus. An outline protocol for haemadsorption is given in *Protocol 4*.

Protocol 4. Protocol for haemadsorption

This is used to detect haemadsorbing (haemagglutinating) viruses producing minimal cytopathic effect in test tube cell cultures.

1. Thoroughly wash a suspension of human group 'O' red blood cells (RBCs) in PBS.
2. Prepare a suspension of 0.4% v/v RBCs in PBS.
3. Remove culture fluid by aspiration with Pasteur pipette and discard into disinfectant solution.
4. Add six drops of RBCs to infected and control tubes with a Pasteur pipette.
5. Spread RBCs over cell sheet and place in incubation rack at 4°C for 20 min.
6. Pour off surplus RBCs, wash twice with PBS, and examine under a microscope without delay.

Individual haemadsorbing viruses can be identified by blocking the haemagglutinins with a suitable antiserum before adding the human group 'O' cells. Absence of haemadsorption relative to controls confirms identity.

Individual viruses can be identified by haemadsorption inhibition, immunofluorescence, or neutralization. As with other aspects of diagnostic virology, the quickest and simplest method is the best. For years, the characteristic pocks on the chorio-allantoic egg membrane were used to distinguish between herpes simplex virus types 1 and 2. This was unsatisfactory as it did not always give a clear result. Immunofluorescence with mAbs is much quicker and more clear-cut (8), while the same technique can be used to identify/distinguish otherwise poorly growing or non-growing adenovirus types 40 and 41 (J. S. M. Peiris, unpublished).

Finally, rhinoviruses may be distinguished from enteroviruses by their sensitivity to low pH in an acid-stability test. The isolate is treated with a buffer at pH 3.0 and the pH re-adjusted to neutrality; the isolate is then tested for survival in further cell cultures. Enteroviruses will survive this treatment, whereas rhinoviruses will not.

Neutralization (*Protocol 5*) is usually necessary for serotype identification, particularly with enteroviruses and adenoviruses. The large number of the former is covered by pools of poliovirus- and coxsackie B virus-specific antisera and the Lim–Benyesh–Melnick intersecting echovirus antibody pools (9). The neutralization test is used to identify individual serotypes of enteroviruses (polioviruses, cultivatable coxsackie A viruses, coxsackie B viruses, echoviruses, adenoviruses, etc.) by mixing specific antisera with virus isolates, and testing the mixture for residual infectivity in a suitable cell culture. The

---

Protocol 5. Protocol for neutralization test

1. Prepare antisera at working dilution[a] in cell culture maintenance medium (as diluent).[b]

2. Dilute virus (isolate) similarly as necessary.[c]

3. Mix 0.1 ml of each antiserum with the same volume of virus in bijou bottles or a multiwell plate.

4. Prepare a control mixture of 0.1 ml virus and 0.1 ml of diluent.

5. Allow to react (covered if on a plate) at room temperature for 1 hour.[d]

6. Inoculate 0.1 ml of each mixture into a suitable cell culture.[e]

7. Include a cell control inoculated with diluent alone.

8. Incubate at 37 °C and read daily until the virus control shows advanced cytopathic effect.[f]

[a] Based on supplier's figures and confirmed by testing on standard virus strains.
[b] Some virologists prefer to use PBS.
[c] Ideally 100 $TCID_{50}$ per 0.1 ml but neutralization is both labour-intensive and expensive. Hence the dilution is usually 1 in 10 or 1 in 100 of the isolate (preferences differ and depend on the stage of CPE when the isolate is harvested for identification). See also footnote f.
[d] The time and temperature of incubating the neutralization mixture varies greatly between laboratories.
[e] In which the putative virus will grow reliably.
[f] Because wild-type viruses do not always passage reliably, virologists prefer to see 'breakthrough' by the virus even where most of the virus is neutralized by a specific serum. Hence a neutralization test should be read at the optimum point when the control cultures and those containing non-neutralizing sera show CPE but the virus had not broken through the neutralizing serum or pool of sera.

---

variety of serotypes frequently makes this a two-stage process in which pooled antisera are first used to identify the virus genus and the serotype in a second test. *Protocol 5* is illustrative; different laboratories develop their own to suit their requirements. Although described here as a test to identify an isolate, the same test can be used to measure antibody by mixing dilutions with standard amounts of virus.

2.5 Animal inoculation

Most coxsackie A viruses and a few others do not grow in cell culture but will grow in newborn mice or other experimental animals. Most laboratories have found the yield of positives to be so low that they are gradually abandoning animal inoculation. As a result, occasional infections will remain undiagnosed.

There has been a similar decline in the use of fertile hen's eggs, once routinely used in most virus laboratories. Some strains of influenza viruses grow poorly in available cell cultures and amniotic inoculation is still used as the last resort. However, the bulky egg incubator now governed in the UK by the Animals (Scientific Procedures) Act of 1986, is being increasingly ignored in its separate room.

The use of other animals in routine laboratories in the UK is very rare. Investigation of new viruses and syndromes may turn the virologist's thoughts towards the animal house from time to time but usually only if other approaches fail. As molecular techniques can by-pass growth of the virus completely, the use of animals in diagnosis will continue to decline, though not, I believe, the use of cell culture.

2.6 Serology

This can be defined as an investigation into whether a patient has mounted an antibody response to one or more viral antigens. It can be used diagnostically in two ways: to assess **serostatus**, i.e. whether an individual has encountered a virus before and is, therefore, presumptively immune, or, by demonstrating evidence of a recent infection (**serodiagnosis**).

2.6.1 Serostatus

This requires a test which detects long-term (usually IgG class) antibody. The timing of serum sampling is not critical for this technique and is determined by other factors, for example, rubella virus antibody screening is performed in early pregnancy and CMV serostatus of donor and recipient in transplant surgery. One specimen will usually be sufficient though a negative CMV result in a patient awaiting a transplant will require further monitoring until the operation takes place.

2.6.2 Serodiagnosis

Here the purpose is to secure evidence of recent viral infection, provided either by seroconversion (appearance of new antibody), a rise in titre, a titre high enough to be unlikely to have been due to infection long ago, or by the presence of IgM class antibody.

i. Seroconversion

This is the most unequivocal evidence. It is defined as absence of antibody at the acute stage of the disease followed by its presence 10–14 days later in the convalescent stage. It requires two specimens of blood (as serum) taken at acute and convalescent stages.

ii. Rising titre

Usually this is defined as an increase of ≥4-fold in titre but it should be defined more correctly as an increase which cannot be due to chance. With most tests (and hence titres) depending on doubling dilution series the 4-fold rise fulfils literally this condition but will require analysis before it is reported (see Section 2.6.4).

iii. High titre

Antibody responses after infection will usually rise to a peak, then fall slightly before levelling out at the titre which will persist. Hence such peak levels are usually taken to indicate a recent infection, though the level taken to be significant will vary with the virus concerned and the test used to detect antibody to it.

iv. IgM antibody

This class of antibody is the body's first response and is mainly produced in response to a primary infection. However, prolonged presence of virus-specific IgM antibodies has been described, so care in interpretation of positive IgM results has to be taken (see below).

2.6.3 Techniques

Considerable ingenuity has been shown in devising tests for measuring antibody levels. In essence, such tests consist of mixing an antigen with the patient's serum and adding an indicator system to show that antibody from the patient has reacted with the antigen. The diversity comes from the need to distinguish true antibody from non-specific inhibitors, to be simple to do, and capable of being applied to as many specimens as required. There is no virtue in listing all variants, but two examples merit a specific mention, one of which will be discussed further in Chapter 2.

Complement fixation tests (CFTs) based on the technique of Bradstreet and Taylor (10) have been the mainstay of diagnostic viral serology in many laboratories for about 30 years despite chronic problems of instability, reproducibility and, frequently, non-specificity. They have maintained their place despite these difficulties for three reasons:

(a) A wide variety of viral antigens prepared for use in CFTs was available free of charge until recently in the UK to diagnostic laboratories through the PHLS. They are of good quality, and many laboratories have come to depend on them.

(b) The test detects short-term antibody so that it is possible to screen the convalescent serum against appropriate antigens and titrate out only those that are positive. Hence most screening tests are negative with potential positives clearly visible against a generally negative background.

(c) In the microtitre format semi-automation is possible.

It is only recently that it has become possible, using genetic engineering, to mass produce antigens for use in commercial kits. This has led to a plethora of new assays, many based on enzyme immunoassays (EIAs) or ELISAs (enzyme-linked immunosorbent assays). Since, using such techniques, it will be more expensive to cover the same spectrum of viruses, the CFT may retain its place for a time but, because it does not detect long-term antibody reliably, it has never had a place in assessing serostatus.

Enzyme immunoassays, particularly capture assays, can assess levels of IgM and IgG antibodies. As such they might have replaced CFTs already had a full range of tested antigens and conjugates been available, but this is not the case and may never be. As capture assays, they are 'cleaner' than CFTs with fewer difficult results. However, as with every test so far devised they have a 'grey' (borderline) zone which will remain despite the most careful assessment of the cut-off level.

Capture assays to indicate recent infection by detecting IgM antibody offer the possibility of confirming the diagnosis on a single sample of serum. The presence of IgM confirms a recent or continuing stimulus but the single serum sample has to be taken sufficiently long after onset (about 1 week minimum for reliability). However, such assays have an increasing value in demonstrating recent, continuing, or renewed virus activity. Examples include hepatitis A and B virus infection, recent rubella virus infection, recrudescence of CMV activity after organ transplantation, Epstein–Barr virus (EBV) infection, etc. It seems unlikely, though, that they will replace completely the traditional use of paired samples of sera. Details of EIAs are presented in Chapter 2.

2.6.2 Interpretation of serological results

Production of antibody confirms a stimulus to the immune mechanisms. It gives no indication of where the stimulus was applied or of what it signifies. The results of a serological test should therefore always carry an interpretation by the virologist.

Compared with isolating the virus, particularly from the affected organ, serology is indirect and the results often too late to influence management, though persistent IgM-class antibody can be a valuable indicator of continuing virus activity. The main exceptions are provided by three agents which are not viruses but are traditionally diagnosed in virology laboratories. Infections with *Mycoplasma pneumoniae*, *Coxiella burnetii* and chlamydiae usually have an insidious onset and protracted course. Antibody levels have often risen by the time diagnosis is attempted and, because treatment is possible, serology is both timely and worthwhile.

Apart from these examples and in assessments of serostatus, serology mainly serves as a back-up to other more rapid techniques. As such it serves a valuable function and is the core of operations in private laboratories which find the costs of the techniques for finding virus unacceptably high. Nonetheless, the main value of serology alone is in confirming what has happened. There are a considerable number of viruses for which serological tests are not available, usually because of multiple serotypes and lack of a group antigen (enteroviruses, other than poliovirus, coxsackie B viruses, and rhinoviruses, for example).

Serological results should always be seen in context and never accepted without considering the circumstances.

3. Developments in diagnosis

Two factors will promote developments in virus diagnosis. Firstly, new drugs for treating virus infections will require cheap reliable tests which are positive early in the disease or, as in transplant patients, before it starts. They are largely available already. The second factor will be increasing cost-consciousness. How the value of diagnosis is assessed in terms of shortening hospital stay, withholding antibiotics, using antiviral agents, and the value of a firm diagnosis cutting out further (expensive) investigations remains to be seen. The need for epidemiological information of virus infections adds to the value of diagnosis.

New developments must include better early diagnosis of infections with human immunodeficiency virus, evaluation of nucleic acid detection techniques such as the polymerase chain reaction (PCR) (see Chapter 5) which may reveal hitherto unrecognized latency by a variety of viruses (with the attendant task of understanding the significance) and filling the gaps in rapid (i.e. same-day) techniques for diagnosis of CMV, enterovirus, and rhinovirus infections. New viruses and associated diseases will bring new diagnostic problems.

The biggest problem will be how to provide diagnosis for all. Diagnostic virology works best over short lines of communication, but it is unlikely, at present, that each District General Hospital will have its own virologist with a dedicated laboratory. Comprehensive diagnostic virology may become largely a regional activity with local microbiology laboratories carrying out mainly kit-based tests. Any problems would be referred to the regional laboratory. This solution will be far from satisfactory. Viruses will not become less important with time, and the District General Hospital virology laboratory may eventually become a necessity.

The remaining chapters in this book will point towards new approaches, some already available and in use in some laboratories, others experimental at present. Against them the traditional techniques discussed above will have to prove their continuing value in providing timely, accurate, and relatively inexpensive answers, but tradition should not be discarded lightly.

References

1. Lin, Y. P., Nicholas, K., Ball, F. R., McLaughlin, B. and Bishai, F. R. (1991). Detection of Norwalk-like virus and specific antibody by immune-electron micro-scopy with colloidal gold immune complexes. *J. Virol. Methods*, **35**, 237–54.
2. Doane, F. W. and Anderson, N. (1987). *Electron microscopy in diagnostic virology*. Cambridge University Press.
3. Palmer, E. L. and Martin, M. L. (1988). *Electron microscopy in viral diagnosis*. CRC Press, Boca Raton, FL.
4. Madeley, C. R. and Field, A. M. (1988). *Virus morphology*, 2nd edn. Churchill Livingstone, Edinburgh.
5. McGuckin, R., and Taylor, C. E. (1995). In *Handbook of diagnostic virology* (ed. J. M. Best, P. Morgan-Capner, J. Bertrand, and J. Foster). Cambridge University Press.
6. Goldwasser, R. A., and Shepard, C. C. (1958). Staining of complement and modifications of fluorescent antibody procedures. *J. Immunol.*, **80**, 122–31.
7. Gardner, P. S. and McQuillin, J. (1980). *Rapid virus diagnosis, application of immunofluorescence*, 2nd edn. Butterworths, London.
8. Gleaves, C. A., Wilson, D. J., Wold, A. D., and Smith, T. F. (1985). Detection and serotyping of herpes simplex virus in MRC-5 cells by use of centrifugation and monoclonal antibodies 16h post-inculation. *J. Clin. Microbiol.* **21**, 29–32.
9. Melnick, J. L. and Wimberly, I. L. (1985). Lyophilized combination pools of enterovirus equine antisera: new LBM pools prepared from reserves stored frozen for two decades. *Bull. WHO*, **63**, 543–50.
10. Grist, N. R., Bell, E. J., Follett, E. A. C., and Urquhart, G. E. D. (1979). *Diagnostic methods in clinical virology*, 3rd edn, pp. 95–115. Blackwell Scientific Publications, Oxford.

2

Immunoassays

J. J. GRAY and T. G. WREGHITT

1. Immunoassays

During the past decade, immunoassays to detect viral antigens and virus-specific antibodies have gained tremendous popularity in clinical laboratories. There are many assay formats available for detecting either viral antigens or antibodies. These may be constructed by attaching either viral antigen, virus-specific antibody, or anti-human class-specific immunoglobulin to the solid phase. An example of this is the indirect antibody assay, where viral antigen is attached to the solid phase. The bound antigen is then used to capture virus-specific antibodies in patients' sera and the presence of the captured antibody is detected with a labelled anti-human antibody. This antibody may be labelled either with enzymes such as horseradish peroxidase or alkaline phosphatase or with a radioisotope such as ^{125}I. Tests for viral antigens are constructed in an analogous way (see below). Enzyme labels offer the advantages of longer shelf-life and easier disposal, and equipment associated with enzyme immunoassays is usually less expensive. In the following we describe different modifications of such test systems.

2. Enzyme-linked immunosorbent assays (ELISAs)

ELISAs are widely used in clinical virology laboratories for detecting viral antigens and antibodies. Enzyme-labelled conjugates are stable, and the test formats are amenable to automation. Assays may be read spectrophotometrically and quantitative results obtained by comparison with standards. Tests can be performed with a minimum of equipment, making them suitable for use even in small virology laboratories.

2.1 Solid phase

Antigen or antibody are passively adsorbed on a solid phase, probably as a result of hydrophobic interactions between molecules of the solid phase and the antigen or antibody. Microtitre plates, beads, tubes, and cuvettes made of polystyrene, polyvinyl, polycarbonate, or nylon may be used as the solid phase in immunoassays. The type of carrier chosen should take into account the instrumentation available. The material used, and its treatment (e.g. gamma-irradiation), should be chosen for its binding capacity and uniformity of binding.

When constructing a new assay, the solid phase should be selected with care. Several batches from different manufacturers should be tested for their suitability. The possibility of inter-batch variation and of differences in binding properties between different wells on the same plate exists.

2.2 Antigen preparation

The majority of viral antigens used in serological tests are produced from infected cell cultures. The cell culture-derived antigens may have to be partially purified before use in enzyme immunoassays (see *Table 1*). In particular, in indirect ELISAs where antigen is bound to the plastic, excessive background reactivity resulting from contamination of the antigen by cell culture components may make the interpretation of results impossible. Where sufficient purification is not possible, a control antigen consisting of

---

Table 1. Preparation of viral antigens for use in ELISAs

Virus	Antigen preparation	Reference
Herpes simplex virus	Grow virus in BHK21 cell culture; solubilize with detergent; purify by ion exchange chromatography	1
Cytomegalovirus	Grow virus in human embryo lung cell culture; extract in alkaline glycine buffer	2
Varicella-zoster virus	Grow virus in human embryo lung cell culture; extract in alkaline glycine buffer	3
Rubella virus	Grow virus in Vero cell culture; extract in alkaline glycine buffer	4
Enterovirus	Grow virus in Vero cell culture; purify by freeze–thaw and centrifugation; use uninfected cells as antigen control	5
Rotavirus	Use bovine rotavirus (faecal extract); treat with arcton and purify by differential and isopycnic ultracentrifugation	6
Hepatitis A virus	Grow virus in continuous primate cell culture; lyse cells and purify by centrifugation	7
Hepatitis B virus	Use HBsAg purified from human plasma or recombinant HBsAg produced in yeast	8
Hepatitis C virus	Recombinant antigen produced in yeast	9
Human immunodeficiency virus	Synthetic peptides or recombinant antigen	10

---

uninfected cells, treated in the same way as the infected cell preparation, should be included in the test.

2.3 Enzyme conjugation

Horseradish peroxidase (HRPO) and alkaline phosphatase (AP) have been extensively used as labels in immunoassays. Methods to conjugate these enzymes with antibodies are outlined in *Protocols 1* and *2*, respectively. There are many methods of conjugation in present use, and the choice of method will depend on the ability of the antibody to conjugate. The efficiency of conjugation of monoclonal antibodies, in particular, can vary. Therefore, if unsuccessful, alternative methods should be tried (11).

Protocol 1. Preparation of HRPO-conjugated antibodies

Equipment and reagents

- CX30 ultrafiltration unit (Millipore)
- Spectrophotometer capable of measuring absorbance at 280 nm and 403 nm
- 100 mM sodium bicarbonate buffer, pH 9.2
- 0.01 M PBS pH 7.2 (Oxoid)

- Sephadex G-25 (Pharmacia Ltd)
- Thiomersal
- Sephacryl S200 (Pharmacia Ltd)
- Affinity purified HRPO (Sigma)

Method

1. Add 5 mg of purified HRPO to 0.5 ml of freshly prepared 100 mM NaHCO$_3$ in a small tube.

2. Add 0.5 ml of 16 mM sodium periodate, close the tube, and incubate at room temperature for 2 h in the dark.

3. Dissolve 15 mg of IgG in 2 ml of 100 mM sodium carbonate buffer pH 9.2.

4. Add the activated HRPO and IgG to a glass-wool-plugged Pasteur pipette (the tip closed by melting).

5. Immediately add dry Sephadex G-25 (one-sixth of the combined weight of enzyme and antibody) and incubate for 3 h at room temperature.

6. Break the end of the Pasteur pipette and elute the conjugate from the Sephadex.

7. Add 1/20th volume of freshly prepared NaBH$_4$ (5 mg/ml in 0.1 mM NaOH) and incubate for 30 min at room temperature.

8. Add 1/10th volume of the NaBH$_4$ solution and incubate for 1 h at 4°C.

9. Reduce the reaction volume to approximately half by dialysis against a saturated solution of sucrose for 1 h at room temperature.

10. Separate the conjugated antibody from unbound HRPO by chromatography on Sephacryl S200 equilibrated with PBS.

Protocol 1. *Continued*

11. Collect 5 ml fractions and measure the absorbance at 280 nm (to detect IgG) and at 403 nm (to detect HRPO).

12. Pool fractions containing both IgG and HRPO.

13. Concentrate the pooled eluate to the original starting volume in a Millipore CX30 ultrafiltration unit.

14. Add Thiomersal to 0.01% final concentration and store the conjugate undiluted at 4 °C.

Protocol 2. Preparation of alkaline phosphatase-conjugated antibodies

Equipment and reagents

- Dialysis tubing
- Alkaline phosphatase (Sigma)
- 20 mM succinimidyl-4-(*N*-maleimido-methyl)-cyclohexane-1-carboxylate (Sigma) in dimethylformamide
- Sephacryl S300 (Pharmacia)
- Dialysis buffer 1: 0.1 M triethanolamine/0.1 M EDTA, pH 7.5

- Dialysis buffer 2: 0.1 M triethanolamine/1 mM $MgCl_2$/0.1 mM ZnCl pH 8.0
- 0.2 M Dithiothreitol (DTT)
- 1 M Tris–HCl, pH 8.0
- 2-Mercaptoethanol
- CX30 ultrafiltration unit (Millipore)
- 0.1% Sodium azide

Method

1. Dialyse 1 ml of purified antibody (1 mg/ml) for 15 h against five 1 litre changes of dialysis buffer 1 at 4 °C with stirring.

2. Add 50 μl of 0.2 M DTT to the dialysed antibody and incubate for 2 h at room temperature.

3. Meanwhile, to a separate vessel, add 200 μl of alkaline phosphatase (10 mg/ml) and 20 μl of 20 mM succinimidyl-4-(*N*-maleimidomethyl)-cyclohexane-1-carboxylate in dimethyl formamide and incubate for 30 min at room temperature. Then add 20 μl of 1 M Tris–HCl pH 8.0.

4. Dialyse both mixtures separately against five 1 litre changes of dialysis buffer 2 for 15 h at 4 °C with stirring.

5. Estimate the volume of enzyme–maleimide retentate and for every 100 μl of enzyme–maleimide add 900 μl of dialysed antibody.

6. Flush the reaction mixture with nitrogen and incubate overnight at 4 °C.

7. Add 2-mercaptoethanol to a final concentration of 50 mM and load the mixture on to a Sephacryl S300 column equilibrated with dialysis buffer 2.

8. Collect and monitor 5 ml fractions at 280 nm and test the fractions showing peak absorbance for conjugate activity.

9. Pool the active fractions, concentrate them in a CX30 ultrafiltration unit (see *Protocol 1*), and store at 4 °C with 0.1% sodium azide preservative.

2.4 Basic assay methods

Indirect, competitive, and antibody-capture ELISAs are commonly used to detect antibody (see *Figure 1*). The choice of assay will be governed by several factors. An indirect assay (see *Protocol 3*) is capable of determining antibody quantitatively but may require purified antigen whereas a competitive

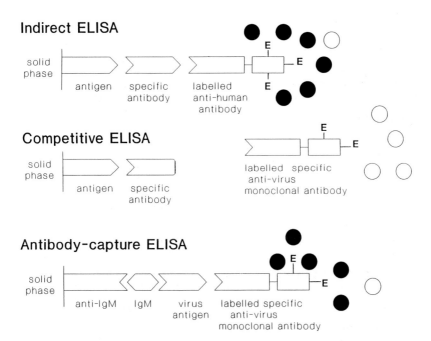

Figure 1. Indirect, competitive, and antibody capture ELISAs. In the indirect ELISA the presence of antibody, complexed with an antigen bound to the solid phase, is detected with an enzyme-labelled anti-human antibody. The bound enzyme, in the presence of the appropriate substrate, will then catalyse the production of a coloured product. In the competitive ELISA a coloured product is not produced since specific antibody, present in the patient's serum, prevents the labelled specific antibody from binding to the antigen. The IgM capture ELISA uses anti-human IgM to capture IgM molecules from the sample. Specific IgM is then detected by adding a specific viral antigen followed by a labelled specific anti-viral antibody. Filled circles, coloured product; open circles, unused substrate.

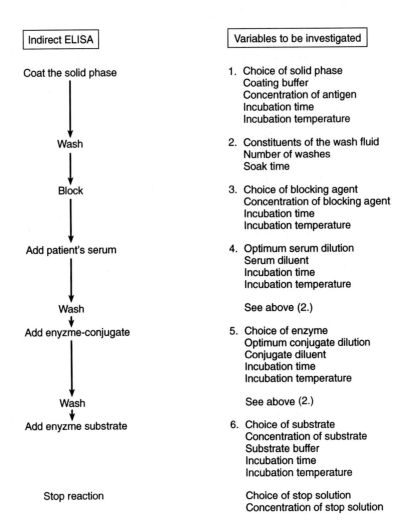

Indirect ELISA	Variables to be investigated

Coat the solid phase

1. Choice of solid phase
   Coating buffer
   Concentration of antigen
   Incubation time
   Incubation temperature

Wash

2. Constituents of the wash fluid
   Number of washes
   Soak time

Block

3. Choice of blocking agent
   Concentration of blocking agent
   Incubation time
   Incubation temperature

Add patient's serum

4. Optimum serum dilution
   Serum diluent
   Incubation time
   Incubation temperature

Wash

See above (2.)

Add enyzme-conjugate

5. Choice of enzyme
   Optimum conjugate dilution
   Conjugate diluent
   Incubation time
   Incubation temperature

Wash

See above (2.)

Add enyzme substrate

6. Choice of substrate
   Concentration of substrate
   Substrate buffer
   Incubation time
   Incubation temperature

Stop reaction

Choice of stop solution
Concentration of stop solution

Figure 2. Variables that need to be investigated when developing an indirect ELISA. (1) The choice of solid phase may be governed by the availability of suitable equipment such as the washer and spectrophotometer. Antigen or antibody to be coated on to the solid phase should be suspended in a suitable buffer e.g. 0.1 M sodium carbonate/bicarbonate buffer pH 9.6. Incubation for 4 h at room temperature or overnight at 4 °C may be used. (2) Five wash cycles with PBS or normal saline containing 0.05% Tween 20 with a soak time of 30 sec is an efficient wash procedure. (3) Blocking can be achieved by adding either PBS containing 0.5% BSA, 5% NRS, or 5% skimmed milk powder and incubating for 1 h at 37 °C or overnight at 4 °C. (4) The optimum serum dilution should be determined and the serum diluent should contain protein, e.g. NRS or fetal calf serum, to prevent the non-specific attachment of antibodies. Incubation for 1–2 h at 37 °C is common in this type of assay. (5) The choice of enzyme may depend on the presence of endogenous enzymes in the antigen preparation. The optimum conjugate dilution should be determined and the diluent should contain protein. Incubation for 1–2 h at 37 °C is common. (6) The choice of substate, optimum concentration, substrate buffer, and stop solution will depend on the enzyme used (see *Table 2*).

assay (see *Protocol 4*) is more suitable for epidemiological studies where the presence or absence of antibody need to be determined (qualititative assay). Although antibody-capture assays (see *Protocol 5*) can be used to detect any class of antibody, they are predominantly used to detect IgM. Indirect and competitive ELISAs are also used to detect virus antigen in clinical samples (see *Protocol 6*).

The optimum concentration of antigen or antibody coated on to the microtitre plate, the optimum dilution of test serum, and the optimum concentrations of enzyme conjugate and enzyme substrate must be determined empirically for each assay system (see *Figure 2*). The choice of enzyme is usually one of convenience but may be influenced by the presence of endogenous enzymes in the antigen or clinical sample (e.g. alkaline phosphatase in faeces). These endogenous enzymes can produce unacceptable background readings. Endogenous alkaline phosphatases may be blocked by adding 20 µl of 1.0 M levamisole to every 10 ml of substrate buffer. Levamisole will block all endogenous alkaline phosphatases except intestinal alkaline phosphatase.

Protocol 3. Indirect ELISA for detecting antibody

Equipment and reagents

- Microtitre plates (flexible; 96 flat-bottomed wells; Becton-Dickinson)
- Spectrophotometer with 405, 450, 492, 510 and 540 nm filters (Flow Laboratories)
- Coating buffer: 0.1 M sodium carbonate/ bicarbonate pH 9.6
- PBST: PBS (see *Protocol 1*) containing 0.05% Tween 20

- Blocking buffer: PBS containing either 0.5% bovine serum albumin (BSA), 5% normal rabbit serum (NRS), or 5% skimmed milk powder
- Enzyme-conjugated anti-human IgM or IgG (Dako) (see *Protocols 1* and *2*)
- Enzyme substrate (see *Table 2*)

Method

1. Coat the wells of a microtitre plate with 100 µl of viral antigen at a predetermined concentration (and alternate wells with uninfected control antigen where appropriate) in coating buffer.

2. Cover the plate and incubate overnight at 4°C overnight in a moist atmosphere.

3. Wash the plate three times with PBST. In each wash, completely fill the empty wells.

4. Block for 30 min at 37°C with 100 µl of PBS containing either 0.5% BSA, 5% NRS, or 5% skimmed milk powder.

5. Remove the blocking agent by aspiration.

6. Add 100 µl of test serum diluted 1 in 100 in PBST (include positive and negative control sera).

7. Incubate at 37°C in a moist atmosphere for 1 h.

Protocol 3. *Continued*

8. Wash the plate five times with PBST.

9. Add 100 μl of enzyme-conjugated anti-human IgM or IgG antibody at a pre-determined dilution (usually between 1 in 1000 and 1 in 5000).

10. Incubate at 37 °C in a moist atmosphere for 1 h.

11. Wash the plate as described in step 3.

12. Add 100 μl of enzyme substrate (see *Table 2*) to each well.

13. Incubate at room temperature for 30 min.

14. Stop the reaction and measure optical density values at specified wavelength (see *Table 2*).

Protocol 4. Competitive ELISA for detecting antibody.

Equipment and reagents

- Microtitre plates (see *Protocol 3*)
- Spectrophotometer (see *Protocol 3*)

- Enzyme-conjugated anti-virus monoclonal antibody (see *Protocols 1* and *2*).
- Enzyme substrate (see *Table 2*)

Method

1. Coat the wells of a microtitre plate with viral antigen as described in *Protocol 3*.

2. Wash the plate and block any unused sites as described in *Protocol 3*, steps 3 and 4.

3. Remove the blocking agent by aspiration.

4. Add 100 μl of undiluted serum (include positive and negative control sera).

5. Incubate at 37 °C in a moist atmosphere for 2 h.

6. Wash the plate five times with PBST (see *Protocol 3*, step 3).

7. Add 100 μl of enzyme-conjugated anti-virus monoclonal antibody at a pre-determined dilution.

8. Incubate for 2 h in a moist atmosphere at 37 °C.

9. Wash the plate as before.

10. Add 100 μl of enzyme substrate (see *Table 2*)

11. Incubate at room temperature for 30 min.

12. Stop the reaction and measure optical density values at specified wavelength (see *Table 2*).

Protocol 5. Antibody-capture ELISA

Equipment and reagents

- Microtitre plates (see *Protocol 3*)
- Spectrophotometer (see *Protocol 3*)
- Anti-human IgM (μ-chain) (Dako)
- Anti-human IgG (γ-chain) (Dako)
- Coating buffer (see *Protocol 3*)
- Blocking buffer (see *Protocol 3*)

- Enzyme-conjugated anti-virus antibody (see *Protocols 1* and *2*)
- Enzyme substrate (see *Table 2*)
- PBST containing 10% fetal bovine serum (FBS)

Method

1. Coat the wells of a microtitre plate with 100 μl of antibody to human IgM (μ-chain) or human IgG (γ-chain) at a pre-determined concentration in coating buffer.

2. Cover the plate and incubate overnight in a moist atmosphere at 4°C.

3. Wash the plate three times with PBST (see *Protocol 3*, step 3).

4. Block for 30 min at 37°C with PBS containing either 0.5% BSA, 5% NRS, or 5% skimmed milk powder.

5. Remove the blocking agent by aspiration.

6. Add 100 μl of test serum diluted 1 in 100 in PBST (include positive and negative controls).

7. Incubate for 2 h in a moist atmosphere at 37°C.

8. Wash the plate five times with PBST as before.

9. Add 100 μl of viral antigen diluted in PBST containing 10% FBS.

10. Incubate overnight in a moist atmosphere at room temperature.

11. Wash the plate five times with PBST as before.

12. Add 100 μl of enzyme-conjugated anti-virus antibody diluted in PBST to a pre-determined dilution.

13. Incubate for 2 h in a moist atmosphere at 37°C.

14. Wash the plate five times with PBST as before.

15. Add 100 μl of enzyme substrate (see *Table 2*) to each well.

16. Incubate for 30 min at room temperature.

17. Stop the reaction and measure optical density values at specified wavelength (see *Table 2*).

Protocol 6. Indirect ELISA for detecting viral antigen

Equipment and reagents

- Microtitre plates (see *Protocol 3*)
- Spectrophotometer (see *Protocol 3*)
- Coating buffer (see *Protocol 3*)
- Blocking buffer (see *Protocol 3*)

- Enzyme-labelled virus-specific antibody (see *Protocols 1 and 2*)
- Enzyme substrate (see *Table 2*)

Method

1. Coat each well of a microtitre plate with 100 µl of a pre-determined concentration of polyclonal or a pool of monoclonal virus-specific antibodies in coating buffer overnight at 4°C.

2. Wash the plate three times with PBST (see *Protocol 3*, step 3).

3. Block for 30 min at 37°C with 100 µl of PBS containing either 0.5% BSA, 5% NRS, or 5% skimmed milk powder.

4. Remove the blocking agent by aspiration.

5. Add 100 µl of cell culture fluid or treated clinical sample (see *Table 3*) to the well and incubate at 37°C for 2 h.

6. Wash the plate five times with PBST as before.

7. Add 100 µl of enzyme-labelled polyclonal virus-specific antibody (produced in a species different from that of the antibody used to coat the plate) or enzyme-labelled monoclonal antibody (directed against different epitopes of the virus) to each well.

8. Incubate at 37°C for 2 h.

9. Add 100 µl of enzyme substrate (see *Table 2*) and incubate for 30 min at room temperature.

10. Stop the reaction and measure the optical density values at specified wavelength (see *Table 2*).

2.5 Enzyme amplification

Enzyme amplification has been employed to increase the sensitivity of ELISAs, particularly those for detecting antigens, which may be present in low concentrations in clinical samples. An example of enzyme amplification, developed by Novo Biolabs, is one in which the bound enzyme catalyses the formation of a second catalyst which produces an amplified colour reaction. An example is shown in *Figure 3* (12).

The avidin–biotin system, which makes use of the high affinity of avidin for biotin, can be used to improve ELISA sensitivity (13). Avidin-or streptavidin-conjugated enzyme labels will attach in high numbers to biotinylated anti-

Table 2. Enzymes conjugated to antibody, their substrates, and parameters to measure products

Enzyme	Substrate or chromogen	Substrate concentration	Stop solution	Wavelength used to measure converted substrate
Alkaline phosphatase	p-nitrophenyl phosphate [a]	1.0 mg/ml	2 M NaOH	405 nm
Glucose oxidase	2,2'-azino-di (3-ethyl-benzothiazoline-6-sulphonate) (ABTS)	0.4 mg/ml and 70 µl 30% hydrogen peroxide/100 ml	1% SDS	405 nm
Horseradish peroxidase	i. ABTS [b]	as above	as above	405 nm
	ii. O-phenylene-diamine (OPD) [c]	1.0 mg/ml and 40 µl 30% hydrogen peroxide/100 ml	2 M sulphuric acid	492 nm
	iii. tetra-methyl-benzidine (TMB) [d]	0.1 mg/ml and 0.014% hydrogen peroxide	2 M sulphuric acid	450 nm
	iv. 5-aminosalicylic acid (5-AS)	1.0 mg/ml and 100 µl 30% hydrogen peroxide/100 ml	3 M NaOH	550 nm
	v. O-dianisidine (3,3'-dimethoxy-benzidine)	0.1 mg/ml	5 M HCl	530 nm
Urease	urea	1.0 mg/ml	1% Thiomersal	450 nm

[a] p-nitrophenyl phosphate substrate buffer pH 9.8: 97 ml diethanolamine, 0.1 g MgCl₂, 800 ml distilled water.
[b] ABTS substrate buffer pH 4.0: 7.19 g Na₂HPO₄, 5.19 g citric acid, made up to 1 litre with distilled water.
[c] OPD substrate buffer pH 5.0: 7.19 g Na₂HPO₄, 5.19 g citric acid, made up to 1 litre with distilled water.
[d] TMB substrate buffer pH 6.0: 8.2 g sodium acetate, 19.21 g citric acid, made up to 1 litre with distilled water.

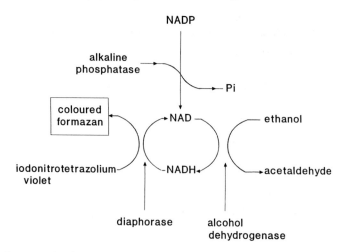

Figure 3. An example of enzyme amplification of substate. NAD, produced from NADP in the reaction catalysed by alkaline phosphatase, is a catalytic activator of a redox cycle which, in the presence of ethanol, alcohol dehydrogenase, and diaphorase, results in iodonitrotetrazolium violet being reduced to the intensely coloured formazan.

body. The high affinity of avidin for biotin results in an increase in the number of enzyme molecules bound and therefore a larger signal is produced in the presence of enzyme substrate.

3. Radioimmunoassay

Radioimmunoassays (RIAs) combine high specificity and sensitivity, but suffer from the short shelf-life of many radiolabelled reagents and from the requirement to comply with regulations governing the safe handling and disposal of radioactive substances. Although, like ELISAs, RIAs can be automated, they are rarely employed in smaller virology laboratories, principally because specimen throughput is insufficient to justify the expense of frequent radiolabelling of reagents or acquisition of commercially produced RIAs.

3.1 Isotopic labels

[125]I, which has a half-life of approximately 60 days, is the most commonly used isotopic label in radioimmunoassays. Alternative isotopes such as ^{35}S, ^{14}C, and ^{3}H have been used but antibodies labelled with ^{35}S may exhibit reduced immunoreactivity and the β-ray-emitting isotopes ^{14}C and ^{3}H involve the use of liquid scintillation counting.

Iodine, when oxidized, will bind to the benzene ring of tyrosine or histidine residues in proteins. Several methods that rely on the oxidation of iodine may be used to produce iodinated antibodies of high specific activity. Among these, treatment with Iodogen (1,2,4,6-tetrachloro-3,6-diphenylglycouracil) produces an iodinated antibody which is highly immunoreactive (see *Protocol 7*).

Protocol 7. Radiolabelling: iodination of IgG

Equipment and reagents

- Gamma counter (Nuclear Enterprises)
- Iodogen (Pierce): 0.5 mg/ml in dichloromethane
- Na^{125}I (Bio-Nuclear Services)
- 0.5 M sodium phosphate buffer pH 7.5 (14.9 g Na$_2$HPO$_4$.2H$_2$O +2.8 g NaH$_2$PO$_4$.2H$_2$O per 200 ml distilled water)
- Saturated potassium iodide in PBS containing 0.1% BSA
- Sephadex G-25 (see *Protocol 1*)
- Elution buffer: PBS containing 0.1% BSA
- 0.01 M PBS

Method

1. Add 20 µl of 0.5 mg/ml Iodogen in dichloromethane to the bottom of an Eppendorf microcentrifuge tube.
2. Dry at room temperature overnight in a fume cupboard.
3. Add 10 µl of 0.5 M sodium phosphate buffer pH 7.5 and 25 µl of IgG (10 µg) to the tube.
4. Add 2.5 ml (0.25 mCi) of Na^{125}I and mix.
5. Incubate for 15 min at room temperature with occasional agitation.
6. Add 500 µl of saturated potassium iodide in PBS containing 0.1% BSA.
7. Load the sample on to a Sephadex G-25 column and wash the sample into the gel with 200 µl of elution buffer.
8. Elute with 1.5–2 column volumes of elution buffer, collecting 20 drop fractions.
9. Estimate the radioactivity of 5 µl aliquots of each fraction in a gamma counter.
10. Pool the fractions collected from the ^{125}I-containing IgG peak and discard free ^{125}I safely.

3.2 Basic assay methods

Indirect and competitive antibody and antigen assays as well as antibody capture assays can be performed by substituting enzyme-labelled with radiolabelled compounds (see *Protocols 3–6*) The more complex washing solutions used in enzyme immunoassays may be replaced with distilled water. If ^{125}I is used, antigen-or antibody-binding is measured with a gamma counter.

4. Luminescence assays

Bioluminescent systems that utilize firefly luminescence, and require the enzyme luciferase, luciferin, magnesium ions, ATP, and molecular oxygen (see *Figure 4*) have been used as alternatives to radiolabels in immunoassays. Luminescence immunoassays combine the specificity of radioimmunoassay with the sensitivity of luminescent light detection. They feature low reagent volumes (and therefore lower cost) and employ stable non-toxic reagents with a shelf-life of around 2 years. The limited availability of reagents such as luciferase has hampered the development of bioluminescent assays.

Chemiluminescence, which uses the phthalhydrazide derivative luminol, hydrogen peroxide, and HRPO (see *Figure 4*), produces low light intensity with rapid decay of light emission. The addition of enhancers such as synthetic luciferin will increase light emission and change the signal from one of short duration, lasting less than 1 sec, to a prolonged output of light lasting several minutes. Detection of emitted light is performed 1–5 min after the addition of substrate (as compared with 20–30 min for ELISA). Therefore enhanced chemiluminescence systems are now incorporated into a wide range of enzyme immunoassays.

4.1 HRPO-catalysed light emission

Assays which use enhanced chemiluminescence systems are constructed and performed in a similar manner to conventional ELISAs (see *Protocols 3–6*).

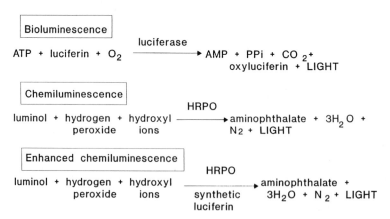

Figure 4. Bioluminescence and chemiluminescence reactions. Bioluminescence reactions are mediated by the bacterial and firefly enzyme luciferase, and involve the oxidation of luciferin to form products including light. Chemiluminescence reactions also involve light production, commonly by oxidation of luminol in the presence of hydrogen peroxide and peroxidase. The reaction may be enhanced by the addition of luciferin, a synthetic component of the firefly bioluminescent system, resulting in a significant increase in peroxidase-catalysed luminescence.

After incubation with the HRPO-conjugated antigen or antibody and normal washing procedures, a solution containing 0.1 M Tris–HC1 pH 8.0, luminol (1.0 mM), luciferin (0.04 mM) or *para*-iodophenol (0.3 mM), and hydrogen peroxide (2.0 mM) is added (14). After 30 sec the light emission is measured by means of a luminometer. The optimum concentration of reagents needs to be determined empirically for each new assay since the activity and concentration of bound HRPO-conjugate will vary.

4.2 Specialized equipment

Chemiluminescence assays require a luminometer in order to measure the signal generated in the assay. The light detection system is stabilized by reference to an internal electrical light source, to compensate for changes in operating temperature and in performance of the detector. If the detector is interfaced with a microcomputer, values for reference reagents can be programmed into the instrument, which may be used to control each assay run by monitoring absolute light levels and comparing expected with actual reference reagent values.

5. Monoclonal antibodies

Antisera produced by immunizing laboratory animals are polyclonal and will contain antibodies with different specificities and affinities as they result from antibody produced by many different lymphocyte clones.

The fusion of terminally differentiated B-lymphocytes with myeloma cells can produce antibody-secreting hybrids, termed hybridomas, which are capable of long-term survival in cell culture (15). The immortalization of antibody-producing cells results in an unlimited supply of antibody with a constant specificity, affinity, and titre.

5.1 Selecting monoclonal antibodies for use in immunoassays

The antigen used to screen for antibody should have undergone the same treatment as that in the immunization protocol, and the immunoassay methodology should be that proposed for the diagnostic test. The ability to screen out low-avidity antibodies should also be incorporated into the assay by use of short incubations or washes with mild detergents such as Tween 20 or by including a mild denaturing agent such as 8 M urea in the wash solution.

6. Evaluation of a commercial immunoassay

Commercial immunoassays should only be introduced into routine use of a laboratory after they have undergone thorough evaluation. This evaluation should determine the test's clinical value with samples collected from the patient population investigated by routine testing. It should, where possible also compare the new test with existing tests and the 'gold standard', i.e. the most sensitive and specific test in current use.

6.1 Selecting samples

Well characterized samples, known to be positive or negative for the specific antigen or antibody and collected from the relevant population, should be included as well as samples which have given equivocal, discordant, or unexpected results. Where available, reference samples calibrated in units of antibody or concentrations of antigen should also be included.

It is important when performing a retrospective study not to exclude patients whose samples gave problems in previous tests as this would bias the result of any evaluation. A prospective study, where samples are tested in parallel with the current assay and the assay being evaluated, protects against biases caused by selecting samples on the basis of results in alternative assays.

6.2 Testing samples

Tests should be performed without knowledge of relevant clinical details or prior laboratory results, and all tests should be carried out under routine conditions. A thorough evaluation of a new commercial immunoassay should consider the test procedures such as sample preparation, incubation times, and equipment required to perform the assay as well as test results.

6.3 Evaluating test performance

Sensitivity, which is the ability of a test to give a positive result for a positive sample, and **specificity**, the ability to identify negative samples correctly, are determined to give a numerical value to the performance of a test. These concepts are defined as:

$$\text{Sensitivity} = \frac{\text{true positives}}{\text{true positives} + \text{false negatives}} \times 100$$

$$\text{Specificity} = \frac{\text{true negatives}}{\text{true negatives} + \text{false positives}} \times 100$$

The **predictive values**, which are the likelihood of a positive result actually being positive and a negative result truly negative are defined as:

$$\text{Positive predictive value} = \frac{\text{true positives}}{\text{true} + \text{false positives}} \times 100$$

$$\text{Negative predictive value} = \frac{\text{true negatives}}{\text{true} + \text{false negatives}} \times 100$$

The predictive value or reliability of a positive or negative result depend on the prevalence in the population of the antigen or antibody detected in the

Table 3. Preparing clinical samples

Sample	Virus detected	Treatment
Cell culture fluid	Herpes simplex virus	Freeze and thaw
Faeces (10% v/v)	Rotavirus; adenovirus	Dilute 1 volume in 4 volumes of PBS containing 0.1 M EDTA
Nasopharyngeal aspirate	Respiratory syncytial virus; influenza A and B viruses; parainfluenza virus; adenovirus	Dilute 1 in 5 in PBS containing 20% fetal calf serum and 2% Tween 20, then sonicate (20 KHz) for 1–2 min

assay. The impact of prevalence can be considered by examining a hypothetical situation where an immunoassay, with a sensitivity of 95.0% and a specificity of 95.0%, for detecting antibody to cytomegalovirus (CMV) is used to study two populations of 1000 people. The prevalence of CMV antibody is 30.0% in a rural population and 80.0% in an urban population. In the population with 30.0% prevalence, 300 people will be antibody-positive and 700 antibody-negative. However, with an assay sensitivity and specificity of 95.0%, only 285/300 antibody-positive and 665/700 antibody-negative samples will be detected, leaving 15 false negative and 35 false positive results. In the population with 80.0% prevalence, 760/800 antibody-positive and 190/200 antibody-negative individuals will be identified correctly, leaving 40 false negative and 10 false positive results. Therefore the reliability of positivity is 89.0% in a population with 30.0% prevalence and increases to 98.7% in a population with 80.0% prevalence. Conversely, the reliability of negativity will be 97.8% in the rural population with 30% antibody prevalence and 82.6% in the urban population with 80% antibody prevalence.

7. Semi-automation and full automation of serological tests

Automation may be introduced into serology laboratories in response to increases in workload. Although the introduction of automated techniques should increase productivity it should also improve the accuracy and reproducibility of any procedure. Many of the procedures associated with immunoassays, including sample preparation, washing, and the addition of reagents, are all suitable for automation.

7.1 Sample dilution

Since the majority of commercial immunoassays are performed in microtitre plates, arranged as eight rows of 12 wells, manufacturers have produced a range of equipment to utilize this format. Multi-channel pipettes, driven by a peristaltic pump such as the Micro-compu pet (General Diagnostics), can be used to pick up and deliver volumes from 5 μl to 9.995 ml.

7.2 Dispensing or reagent addition

Automatic pipetters, ranging from 8-channel to 96-channel, for dispensing reagents into microtitre plates, are widely available. The performance of 96-channel automatic pipetters will be more difficult to monitor and will therefore require more maintenance than an 8-channel machine.

7.3 Plate washing

Washing is an important factor in any solid-phase immunoassay. Insufficient washing will produce high and variable background readings whereas overwashing may decrease the sensitivity of the assay by removing material bound to the solid phase. Appropriate washing cycles for each new assay must be carefully determined. Some assays have very stringent washing requirements.

It is important to ensure that any automated or semi-automated washer fills each well with wash fluid, empties the wells between washes, and performs the appropriate number of washes. The washer should be easily maintained so that wash heads and aspirators are not blocked by crystalline deposits. The plate should be visible throughout the washing procedure. Automated washers should be easily programmable, able to store those programmes, and adaptable to 8-and 12-way microtitre plate formats.

7.4 Reading

Gamma counters, spectrophotometers, and luminometers are an integral part of any automated immunoassay system. Results (which are normally expressed as c.p.m., absorbance values, or photon counts) may be expressed as positive, equivocal, or negative, concentrations of antigen (ng/ml) or international units/litre (IU/litre) of antibody when standards are included in the assay and the equipment is interfaced with a microcomputer.

Equipment should be properly maintained and the efficiency of detectors routinely monitored as part of a quality assurance programme.

7.5 Robotics

A new generation of liquid handling devices, characterized by computer control, high precision, and versatility, has been developed by several commercial companies. Machines such as the Kemble Star 700 Sample Processor have a robotic arm which is directed to move to specific x, y, and z coordinates by the computer programme. This programme may be stored in the computer, thus allowing the procedure to be repeated whenever the programme is recalled. Probes equipped with liquid sensing by means of conductivity measurement enable the machine to dispense, dilute, and wash with great accuracy (16).

Although it is possible to automate immunoassays with this technology, it is difficult to provide a definitive list of manufacturers in such a rapidly evolving area. An enzyme immunoassay, with a protocol stipulating room temperature incubations, and performed on the BIOMEK 1000 (Beckman) which has an inbuilt spectrophotometer, may be completely automated.

8. Quality assurance

The introduction of any new immunoassay into routine use in the laboratory should be accompanied by a quality assurance scheme. The scheme, devised to ensure that any results obtained in the assay are reliable and reproducible, should also be able to pinpoint the cause of any failure in the assay system.

8.1 Source of errors

Potential errors associated with immunoassays, and procedures to limit those errors are summarized in *Table 4*. Operator errors are random and can be kept within acceptable limits only if staff are adequately trained, have an understanding of the assay procedures, and are provided with suitable working conditions.

The incubation conditions, time, temperature, and method of incubation under which an assay is performed should be standardized and limits set. If the assay is performed in microtitre plates, an even temperature can be maintained by placing the plate in a closed box or bag inside the incubator. If a heating block or water bath is used, it is important to ensure that all wells are in contact with the metal or water.

A wide range of equipment may be used during the performance of an immunoassay. Multi-channel pipetters, plate washers, and readers such as spectrophotometers, gamma counters, and luminometers (see Section 7) all

---

Table 4. Common sources of error in immunoassays

Source of error	Procedures to limit error
Operator	Provide adequate training
Incubation conditions	Set parameters for time and temperature of incubation (e.g. 37 °C ± 1 °C for 30 min ± 2 min)
Equipment	Proper maintenance and monitoring
Reagents	Do not mix reagents from different commercial batches Include reagent controls as well as positive and negative controls
Standards	Choose appropriate controls to cover the full working range of the assay

---

have inbuilt errors. The accuracy of spectrophotometers and gamma counters which use multiple detectors depends on the equivalence of the detectors. A quality assurance scheme must include procedures to check the efficiency and equivalence of detectors as any variation may not be detected during routine use. *Table 5* shows results obtained during routine checks on a 16-detector gamma counter. A 30 nCi source was counted for 16 min in each detector. Although the use of appropriate and well-maintained equipment should provide reproducible results, the operator must not assume that results obtained in semi-automated or automated systems are less prone to errors than manual proce-dures. Some of the problems that arise with equipment are listed in *Table 6*.

Reagents provided as part of a commercial immunoassay kit should be used according to the manufacturer's instructions and those from one batch should not be used in another. Reagents produced for 'in-house' assays should be optimized and subsequent batches standardized against the previous batch or known standards. The use of substitute reagents or equipment should be avoided. This procedure, often used as a cost-cutting exercise, may alter the assay performance.

8.2 Controls and standards

Conjugate and substrate controls in enzyme immunoassays and controls to

Table 5. Detector equivalence in a 16-detector gamma counter

| Detector | Test 1 | | Test 2 | |
	Background count	Test count	Background[a] count	Test count
1	680	1 098 309	592	1 103 208
2	712	1 096 836	888	1 099 114
3	656	1 098 955	600	1 106 200
4	424	1 090 097	448	1 100 742
5	512	1 097 616	512	1 073 195
6	488	1 085 765	408	1 098 124
7	432	1 088 614	408	1 101 771
8	560	1 089 266	464	1 101 301
9	824	1 093 134	648	1 103 987
10	400	1 090 569	512	1 099 981
11	544	1 090 183	344	1 103 683
12	624	1 088 582	496	801 614
13	560	1 088 193	536	1 104 701
14	568	1 086 574	592	1 103 147
15	584	1 090 102	416	1 103 016
16	616	1 088 749	552	1 105 039

Test 1: Range, 1 085 765 to 1 098 955; spread, 1.5%
Test 2: Range 801 614 to 1 106 200; spread, 27.8%.
[a] Note that the background count does not detect the faulty detector (number 12) in Test 2.

Table 6. Common faults seen with equipment used in immunoassays

Equipment	Problem	Comment	Solution
Pipetters	Poor calibration	The use of poorly maintained multi-channel pipetters can lead to variations in the volume dispensed from each channel	Maintain multi-channel pipetters and ensure disposable tips are firmly attached
Incubator/water bath	Reduction in assay sensitivity	The assay is optimized at a specific temperature; any change may effect the sensitivity of the assay	Check the temperature of incubator or water bath
	Edge effect [a]	A temperature gradient has been set up across the plate	Incubate in a closed box or bag
Plate washer	Inadequate washing of some wells	The dispensing manifold may become clogged with crystallized wash buffer	Rinse through with distilled water at the end of each day
	Instantaneous colour change after the addition of enzyme substrate	Poor aspiration of the wash fluid	Increase vacuum pressure and tap the plate on an absorbent surface to remove residual wash solution
Gamma counter	High background counts	Radioactive material on the outside of the reaction vessel has contaminated the carrier	Perform counts with empty carrier and discard if contaminated
Spectrophotometer	Low readings	Wrong filter used	Check filter
	Variable readings	Detectors contaminated with dust or damaged by volatile acids used to stop enzyme reactions	Clean or replace detectors
		Condensation on the plate	Wipe the under surface of the plate

[a] Increased or decreased substrate colour development at the edge of the microtitre plate.

determine the efficiency of reagents labelled with radioisotopes are necessary for monitoring the stability of reagents.

Standard serum controls with known antibody titres or containing a specified concentration of antibody should be included in all antibody assays and standard antigen controls with a specified concentration of antigen in all assays to detect antigen. A minimum of three standards should be used and include a strong positive, one low positive or weakly reactive, and at least one (preferably three) negative controls. The low positive control is used to differentiate between positive and negative samples (cut-off control) and will detect any loss of sensitivity in the assay. An alternative method is to employ a series of standards that can be used to construct a dose–response curve. The advantage of this method over the use of a 'cut-off' control is that small changes in the assay conditions will not affect the reproducibility of results. Results obtained with standards, supplied as a component of a commercial immunoassay, should lie within the limits stipulated by the manufacturer. When control values lie outside set limits the results should be rejected, the immunoassay procedures reviewed, and the assay repeated.

8.3 Statistics

The statistical analysis of results obtained in a single immunoassay or collected over a longer period is essential in quality assurance. The arithmetic mean and standard deviation (SD) of each control are calculated from values obtained from at least 20 test runs and if subsequent values lie outside $\pm$ 3SD, the test is 'out of control' and should be checked and remedied.

A number of negative samples (three or more), treated in the same way as the test samples, is included in many immunoassays to establish a mean value for the background signal. This value may be used to select a suitable cut-off value for use in the assay. The choice of cut-off value should be determined by the need to minimize the number of false-positive or false-negative results in any particular assay. For example, immunoassays to detect HBsAg or human immunodeficiency virus antibody in blood donations should have the cut-off value set at a level that would minimize the number of false-negative results so as to avoid transfusion-acquired infection.

Inter-assay variations from day to day can be monitored by calculating the ratio of positive to negative controls. Plotting this value over time will give a crude reflection of changing sensitivity. By this means, progressive changes in assay performance can be detected and remedied.

References

1. Vestergaard, B. F., Grauballe, P. C., and Spangaard, H. (1977). *Acta Pathol. Microbiol. Scand. B*, **85**, 466–8.
2. Betts, R. F., George, S. D., Rundell, B. B., Freeman, R. B., and Douglas, R. G., Jr (1976). *J. Clin. Microbiol.*, **4**, 151–6.

3. Meurisse, E. V. (1969). *J. Med. Microbiol.*, **2**, 317–25.
4. Stewart, G. L., Parkman, P. D., Hopps, H. E., Douglas, R. D., Hamilton, J. P., and Myer, H. M., Jr (1967). *N. Engl. J. Med.*, **276**, 554–7.
5. Muir, P. (1990). In *ELISA in the clinical microbiology laboratory* (ed. T. G. Wreghitt and P. Morgan-Capner), pp. 98–109. PHLS, London.
6. Beards, G. M. (1990). In *ELISA in the clinical microbiology laboratory* (ed. T. G. Wreghitt and P. Morgan-Capner), pp. 110–25. PHLS, London.
7. Hughes, J. V., Stanton, L. W., Tomassini, J. E., Long, W. J., and Scolnick, E. M. (1984). *J. Virol.*, **52**, 465–73.
8. Valenzuela, P., Medina, A., Rutter, W. J., Ammerer, G., and Hall, B. D. (1982). *Nature*, **298**, 347–50.
9. Choo, Q.-L., Kuo, G., Weiner, A. J., Overby, L. R., Bradley, D. W., and Houghton, M. *Science*, **244**, 359–61.
10. Sattentau, Q. J., Dalgleish, A. G., Weiss, R. A., and Beverley, P. C. L. (1986). *Science*, **234**, 1120.
11. Connor, N. S. (1990). In *ELISA in the clinical microbiology laboratory* (ed. T. G. Wreghitt and P. Morgan-Capner), pp. 22–35. PHLS, London.
12. Gatley, S. (1986). *Med. Lab. World*, **43**, 27–8.
13. Guesdon, J. L., Ternynck, T., and Avrameas, S. (1979). *J. Histochem. Cytochem.*, **27**, 1131–9.
14. Whitehead, T. P., Thorpe, G. H. G., Carter, T. J. N., Groucutt, C., and Kricka, L. J. (1983). *Nature*, **305**, 158–9.
15. Kohler, G. and Milstein, C. (1975). *Nature*, **256**, 495–7.
16. Amphlett, M., Smith, D. J., and Warren, R. E. (1991). *J. Med. Microbiol.*, **35**, 249–54.

3

Nucleic acid detection

JONATHAN P. CLEWLEY

1. Introduction

All viruses contain either an RNA or a DNA genome which can be detected
with a suitably designed and prepared complementary probe. Specific binding
of the probe to the target is accomplished by adjusting the stringency—
temperature, salt concentration, and/or formamide concentration—of the
hybridization and post-hybridization washing conditions. The probe is usually
tagged with a radioactive tracer, with a hapten such as biotin or digoxygenin
or with an enzyme such as alkaline phosphatase. The signal from the tracer is
captured on X-ray film or developed as coloured substrate on a solid phase. It
is sometimes possible to quantify this signal to give an estimate of the number
of virus genomes present in the sample. There is an absolute limit of sensitivity of direct hybridization of 10^4–10^5 molecules, depending on the size of the
target genome. At present direct hybridization with ^{32}P-labelled probes of
high specific activity is probably the most sensitive detection method,
although detection by chemiluminescence can be equally sensitive (1). Much
effort has been expended to find ways of increasing the sensitivity of hybridization assays. There are two main approaches to this problem: amplification
of the detection system, or amplification of the target. The sensitivity of the
detection system can be increased by binding multiple probes to the target
(the 'Christmas tree' approach) or by using enzyme cascades (2,3). The DNA
or RNA can be amplified by growing the virus in tissue culture before
hybridization, by concentrating the virus from the sample, or by enzymatic
amplification, of which the polymerase chain reaction (PCR) is the obvious
choice (See Chapter 5).

This chapter does not consider the theory of hybridization, treatments of
which can be found elsewhere (4–6). Methods that have been proven to work
in the laboratories of the author and colleagues are detailed. There are many
variations on protocols from laboratory to laboratory, and many alternative
methods for achieving the same end. Commercial companies supply many
components and kits that can be used in place of home-prepared reagents.
These include complete kits for the hybridization detection of viruses, off-the-
shelf probes, cloning kits, and labelling and hybridization reagents. These

take much of the drudgery out of routine work and, where appropriate, may as well be used.

DNA or RNA hybridization provides direct evidence for the presence of viral genomes in a clinical or pathological specimen, and can be used for diagnosis or for research purposes. Alternatives such as electron microscopy and antigen immunoassay may be less sensitive, but are valuable confirmatory and complementary methods. Growth of virus in tissue culture may not be feasible or may be too time consuming to be of diagnostic use. There are other markers for some viruses, the reverse transcriptase activity of retro-viruses for example, which can be used to show the presence of virus. Obviously, these markers need to be considered in conjunction with the antibody status (specific IgM, IgA, and IgG) of the patient.

Examples of viruses for which a direct, routine hybridization test is useful are human parvovirus B19, hepatitis B virus (HBV), and the human papillo-maviruses (HPVs). The viraemia of human parvovirus B19 precedes the onset of symptoms of disease and antibody response, and is usually intense and short-lived. DNA hybridization is the most appropriate method for detecting virus in specimens suspected of harbouring virus (7). It is also a good method of screening blood donations to find a source of virus for the establishment of serological tests and for cloning viral DNA. DNA hybridization for the detection of HBV in blood and serum is likewise a useful laboratory test, which can be taken as a marker of infectivity instead of e-antigen detection (8). However, in comparison with B19, the amount of circulating HBV is likely to be low and PCR may be a more appropriate method for detecting virus. The HPVs were largely detected and characterized by molecular methods, and typing and diagnosis of the types implicated in genital carcino-mas has been widely used (9).

2. Preparation

Many different types of specimen may be submitted to a diagnostic laboratory for testing for virus. These include serum, plasma and whole blood, tissue, urine, faeces; ceretrospinal fluid (CSF), and nasopharyngeal aspirates (NPA). When planning to test these for viral DNA and RNA, thought should be given to the likelihood that the virions will survive transportation intact. Lysis of an enveloped virus by osmotic or temperature shock will almost certainly result in degradation of a single-stranded (ss) RNA genome. Unfortunately, the best method of preparation of such specimens, i.e. snap freezing and trans-port on dry ice, is often impractical. An alternative is to add a ribonuclease (RNase) inhibitor to the specimen at the time of collection, and to transport it rapidly on wet ice. For instance, 10 mM vanadyl-ribonucleoside complex (VRC; New England Biolabs) could be added to the specimen (10). On arrival in the laboratory the specimen is usually stored frozen or sometimes kept at 4 °C. To minimize RNA (and DNA) degradation it is preferable to process the specimen immediately.

For application of the specimen to a nylon or nitrocellulose filter for dot or slot blotting it may be possible to combine 10–100 μl with 100 μl 2 M NaCl, 1 M NaOH (denaturing solution), and pass this through the membrane using a 96-well microfiltration apparatus (see below). However, if the membrane clogs up, DNA must be extracted from the specimen before application to the filter. Virus can be pelleted by ultra-centrifugation from some specimens, for example urine, before DNA is extracted. Alkaline denaturation is unsuitable for RNA viruses, as RNA is degraded by alkali and binds poorly to membranes under conditions suitable for DNA (see below).

Analysis of the DNA/RNA of some viruses, particularly those that are lymphotropic, is facilitated by the initial purification of peripheral blood mononuclear cells (PBMCs). There are several ways of preparing lymphocytes from whole blood or plasma as described in *Protocols 1–3* below. Blood should preferably be collected into vacutainers containing EDTA (K_3 7.5%, Becton-Dickinson) as heparin can inhibit some nucleic acid detection procedures, for instance PCR.

Protocol 1. Preparation of PBMC from plasma

1. Stand whole blood (2.5 ml) at room temperature for 1.5–2 h, by which time the plasma and erythrocyte fractions will have separated.

2. Remove the plasma carefully, using a fine-tipped plastic pasteur pipette to minimize erythrocyte contamination. Transfer to a 1.5 ml screw-capped tube and adjust the volume to 1 ml with PBS-A (i.e. phosphate-buffered saline without Ca^{2+} or Mg^{2+}), and pellet the cells by centrifuging for 2 min in a microcentrifuge.

3. Discard the supernatant and resuspend the cells in 250 μl PBS-A or H_2O.

4. The cells can be dot blotted, or DNA/RNA can be extracted from them for Southern/Northern analysis.

Although this method is very simple, cell recoveries are variable and highly dependent on the nature of the blood. The method is unsuitable for infant blood and for blood which has been stored for more than 12 h.

Protocol 2. Preparation of lymphocytes by micro-Ficoll gradient centrifugation (11)

1. Carefully layer 0.5 ml of PBS-A over 0.5 ml of Ficoll-Paque (Pharmacia) and add 0.5 ml of EDTA-treated whole blood.

Protocol 2. *Continued*

2. Spin in microcentrifuge for 1 min only and remove layer containing lymphocytes (about 400 μl) with a fine-tipped plastic Pasteur pipette.

3. Pool lymphocytes from two fractions (i.e. 1.0 ml of blood). Top up with PBS and mix thoroughly. Spin in microcentrifuge for 5 min to pellet cells.

4. The cells can be lysed in 90 μl H_2O and dot blotted, or DNA/RNA can be extracted from them for Southern/Northern analysis.

This method can only be used on whole blood which is less than 24 h old, and non-haemolysed. It does not work very well on infant blood.

Protocol 3. Preparation of CD4$^+$ cells with immunomagnetic beads

Equipment and reagents

- Magnetic immunobeads coated with anti-CD4 antibodies (Dynabeads; Dynal)
- Large and small magnetic particle separators (MPC; Dynal)
- 10 ml screw-caped tubes Sterilin, 1.5 ml screw-capped Eppendorf tubes
- PBS-A containing 0.3% BSA

Specimen

Whole blood drawn into EDTA-treated vacutainers. Blood may be stored at 4 °C for up to 24 h before use.

Method

1. Dilute 2 ml of blood with 2 ml ice-cold PBS-A, 0.3% BSA. Blood should preferably be processed within 24 h, but it may be stored for up to 7 days at 4 °C. Add 35 μl of Dynabeads. The bead stock suspension is usually at a concentration of approximately 1.4×10^8/ml (stored at 4 °C and resuspended before use) and should exceed the estimated number of CD4$^+$ cells by approximately 10-fold.

2. Attach the tubes to a rotary mixer and mix gently for 2 h at 4 °C.

3. Transfer the tubes to the larger MPC and stand for 10 min. Without removing the tube, pour off the diluted blood, leaving the pellet of beads and CD4$^+$ cells behind.

4. Wash the beads twice with ice-cold PBS-A/BSA and transfer them to a 1.5 ml Eppendorf tube.

5. Wash again twice, recovering the beads and cells each time by standing the tube in the small MPC for 2 min. After the final wash, add 250 μl ice-cold PBS-A/BSA and mix.

6. The cells can be lysed in and dot blotted, or DNA/RNA can be extracted from them for Southern/Northern analysis.

Chromosomal DNA can be extracted from lymphocytes by the procedure of *Protocol 4*, which is used to extract high molecular weight DNA from virus-infected tissue culture cells. For lymphocytes the procedure is scaled down to 1/10 volume in a microcentrifuge tube, starting at step 2 by resuspending lymphocytes from 0.5 ml of blood in 0.5 ml of lysis buffer. There are about 3.75×10^6 white blood cells per 0.5 ml of blood from a healthy individual.

Protocol 4. High molecular weight DNA preparation from tissue culture cells

1. Trypsinize and spin down (for 10 min at 4 °C in a bench centrifuge) the cells from two 750 ml flasks. Resuspend the cells in PBS and spin them down again.

2. Resuspend the cells in 5 ml of DNA lysis buffer: 50 mM NaCl, 1 mM EDTA, 10 mM Tris-HCl pH 7.4, 2% SDS. Break up the pellet with a cut-off Pasteur pipette, or a cut-off 1 ml micropipette tip. Incubate on ice for 5 min.

3. Add proteinase K (Boehringer Mannheim) to 150 μg/ml and shake at 50 °C for 3 h or 37 °C overnight.

4. Extract three times with phenol/chloroform/isoamyl alcohol (49:49:2, by volume), saturated in TE buffer (20 mM Tris–HCl pH 7.4, 2 mM EDTA) and once with chloroform/isoamylalcohol (49:1; v/v)

5. Add 1/10 volume of 3 M sodium acetate and 2.5 volumes of ethanol. Spool out the DNA with a sealed Pasteur pipette or capillary.

6. Wash the DNA twice by dipping the Pasteur pipette or capillary in 70% ethanol for 2 min.

7. Scrape the DNA into an Eppendorf tube and allow the excess ethanol to evaporate at 37 °C or under vacuum, but do not allow the DNA to dry out completely. Add 0.5 ml of TE buffer and allow the DNA to rehydrate at 4 °C overnight.

The procedure outlined in *Protocol 5* is useful for the extraction of DNA from viruses that replicate in the cytoplasm, e.g. the papovaviruses.

Protocol 5. Extraction of extrachromosomal DNA (12)

1. Decant the medium from the cells grown in the equivalent of a 75 cm^2 flask and add 4 ml of 0.6% SDS in TE buffer (*Protocol 4*). Leave for 20 min at room temperature with occasional rocking for cell lysis to occur. Pour the viscous lysate into a Corex (Du Pont) or Sarstedt tube.

2. Add 1/4 volume of 5 M NaCl. Mix gently and leave at 4 °C for 6 h to overnight.

3. Spin at 10 000 *g* for 15 min in a Sorvall SS-34 rotor or equivalent and collect supernatant.

4. Add an equal volume of phenol equilibrated in TE buffer. Mix and spin for 10 min. Collect the upper phase, add 1/10 volume of 5 M NaCl and 2–3 volumes of absolute ethanol, and leave at −2 °C.

5. Pellet the DNA at 10 000 *g* for 15 min and resuspend in TE buffer.

6. The DNA can be used for dot or slot blotting at this stage; if it is to be analysed by restriction enzyme digestion and Southern blotting further purification may be necessary, as follows.

7. Add the DNA in TE buffer to 3.7–3.8 g of CsCl, 0.25 ml of 2.4 mg/ml ethidium bromide, and adjust the volume to 4 ml. Measure the refractive index (RI) of this solution with a refractometer, and add solid CsCl until the RI is 1.39. Spin at 150 000 *g* in a Beckman SW-50 rotor (or equivalent) for 68 h at 15 °C.

8. Collect the lower band containing the plasmid with a syringe and needle through a side puncture, or with a fine-tipped plastic Pasteur pipette from the top. (The upper band is chromosomal DNA.)

9. Remove the ethidium bromide by washing with 0.5 volumes of isoamyl alcohol until the lower (aqueous) phase is clear. Add three volumes of H$_2$O and to this final volume add a further 2.5 volumes of ethanol. Mix and leave at −20 °C for 2 h to overnight.

10. Recover the DNA by spinning at 10 000 *g* (Sorvall) for 15 min. Discard the supernatant, wash the pellet with 70% ethanol, dry, and resuspend in TE buffer.

Alternatively, whole DNA/RNA can be extracted by a modification of standard proteinase K digestion and phenol/chloroform extraction procedures (*Protocol 6*).

There are many different protocols for the extraction of DNA and RNA from tissues using proteinase K and phenol/chloroform. A simple Tris/NaCl/EDTA/SDS buffer is sometimes used, with incubation from 37 to 55 °C from 1 h to overnight. Sequential extractions with phenol alone, phenol/chloroform, and chloroform alone can be used. The number of extractions, and back extractions of the organic phase with buffer, depends on the nature of the specimen and the judgement of the worker. After the initial phenol/chloroform extractions RNA can be removed, if desired, by the addition of DNase-free RNase at 10–50 μg/ml and incubation at 37°C for 15 min. proteinase K is then added to 100 μg/ml and SDS to 1% and the incubation continued for 30 min at 37°C. The proteinase K can be inactivated by incubation at 95°C for 10–15 min. The residual protein is removed by one phenol/chloroform extraction and one chloroform/isoamyl alcohol extraction, and the DNA is recovered by ethanol precipitation. Different protocols use different salts in the ethanol precipitation step: final concentrations of 0.4 M NaCl, 0.25 M sodium acetate, or 3.75 M ammonium acetate. The latter preferentially precipitates longer pieces of DNA, leaving nucleotides and short oligonucleotides in the supernatant. The time and temperature at which the ethanolic solution is kept before centrifugation also varies. High concentrations of DNA/RNA of high molecular weight will precipitate almost immediately at room temperature. The recovery of low concentrations of DNA/RNA is better if the ethanolic solution is chilled, so long as its viscosity does not impede pelleting of the nucleic acid. An inert carrier such as 100–200 μg of nuclease-free glycogen (Boehringer Mannheim) can be added to co-precipitate small amounts of DNA/RNA. Alternatively, an equivalent amount of tRNA may be used. DNA can also be precipitated by the addition of an equal volume of isopropanol in the presence of 0.5 M ammonium acetate. There are several commercial kits available for extraction of RNA from cells and tissues. These often use a chaotropic agent such as guanidinium isothiocynanate or sodium iodide to disrupt cells and inhibit RNases (see below). It is advisable to consult the catalogues of suppliers of molecular biology reagents to find details of the most recent methods—a quality controlled kit may give better RNA recovery than an in-house method.

Protocol 6. Proteinase K and phenol/chloroform extraction of DNA or RNA

Reagents

- DNA extraction buffer 2× [a]: 8 M urea, 0.4 M NaCl, 0.2 M Tris–HCl pH 8.0, 1% *n*-laurylsarcosine, 0.02 M CDTA (1,2-diaminocyclohexane-tetraacetic acid)

- RNA extraction buffer 10×: 5% SDS, 4 M NaCl, 0.1 M CDTA, 0.5 M Tris–HCl pH 7.4, 1% β-mercaptoethanol

Method

1. For a DNA virus, combine the sample with an equal volume of the 2 × urea buffer. For an RNA virus add 0.1 volume of the RNA extraction buffer and adjust the volume with diethylpyrocarbonate (DEPC) treated H₂O. Extreme precautions must be taken when working with RNA to avoid degradation by nucleases. All solutions must be autoclaved

---

Protocol 6. *Continued*

where possible in water treated with 0.1% DEPC. Mercaptoethanol is not autoclavable. See Sambrook *et al.* (10) for more information on working with RNA. Various RNase inhibitors can be used: for inclusion in enzyme reactions recombinant placental RNasin from Promega is recommended; for addition to clinical specimens a final concentration of 10 mM vanadyl-ribonucleoside complex (VRC) from New England Biolabs is recommended. VRC will inhibit enzyme reactions, but it is usually removed during standard RNA purification procedures.

2. Add proteinase K (Boehringer Mannheim) to 100 µg/ml final concentration (from a 10 mg/ml stock) and incubate at 55 °C for 1 h.

3. Add an equal volume of phenol/chloroform/isoamyl alcohol (49:49:2 by volume, saturated in TE buffer) or 70:30 phenol:chloroform (Applied Biosystems). Mix, spin, and retain the upper aqueous phase.

4. If necessary (if there has been poor phase separation, with a large interface or 'SDS cage') add an equal volume of TE buffer (*Protocol 4*) to the phenol phase and re-extract, mix, and spin. Combine the aqueous phases.

5. Extract the combined aqueous phases with chloroform/isoamyl alcohol (49:1; v/v) by mixing and spinning.

6. Retain the final aqueous phase and add 0.5 volumes of 7.5 M ammonium acetate, and to the resulting total volume add 2 volumes of absolute ethanol for DNA or 2.5 volumes for RNA. Chill at −20 °C for 2 h to overnight and pellet the DNA/RNA by centrifugation. This will usually be with a microcentrifuge for 10–15 min at 11 000 *g*, or with a Sorvall or equivalent centrifuge for 30 min.

7. If the DNA/RNA has been pelleted in 15 or 30 ml Corex tubes, ressolve it in 200 µl of TE buffer, add 100 µl of 7.5 M ammonium acetate and 700 µl of absolute ethanol in a microcentrifuge tube. Chill, spin, wash the pellet with 70% ethanol, and resuspend it in sterile H$_2$O.

a This buffer is as used in the Applied Biosystems DNA extraction machine.

Advances in molecular biology have made DNA analysis of archival material a practical proposition. This may be by dot or Southern blotting, or by PCR. Often stored tissue will be available as paraffin sections, and DNA must be extracted from them before it can be used in hybridization assays or amplified by PCR. An extraction procedure from paraffin blocks is described in *Protocol 7*.

For these protocols it is assumed that the DNA recovered is to be used for dot hybridization, and so no effort is made to remove residual salt and organic solvents. It is necessary to remove these if the DNA is to be digested with restriction enzymes prior to Southern blotting, and if the quality of the DNA is to be assessed spectrophotometrically. To achieve this, extract the final aqueous phase with chloroform/isoamyl alcohol (49:1 (v/v) in TE buffer) before ethanol precipitation, and wash the final DNA pellet with 70% ethanol. The concentration of DNA in the presence of contaminants can be determined using a Hoeffer fluorimeter. Also, if the DNA is to be digested with restriction enzymes, removal of RNA by digestion with DNase-free RNase (e.g. from Promega or Stratagene) may be necessary. This can be achieved by adding the RNase to 20 μg/ml and incubating for 15 min at 37 °C. The RNase can be removed afterwards by proteinase K digestion for 30 min followed by phenol/chloroform extraction and ethanol precipitation.

Protocol 7. Extraction of DNA from paraffin blocks[a]

A. *For large sections*

1. Add a portion of the paraffin block to 2 ml of TE buffer (*Protocol 4*), 0.2 ml of 10% SDS, and 2 ml of phenol/chloroform/isoamyl alcohol (49:49:2 by volume, saturated in TE buffer) in a 15 ml glass Corex tube or a plastic Sarstedt tube. Mix and incubate at 60 °C for 15 min. [Parafilm cannot be used to cover the top of Corex glass tubes as phenol/chloroform dissolves it. Be wary of pressure building up in the Sarstedt tubes if caps are used with them. Adhere to your laboratory's recommended safety procedures for handling and disposal of organic reagents.]

2. Spin at up to 10 000 *g* for 5 min to separate the phases and collect and retain the top aqueous phase.

3. Re-extract the lower organic phase with 2 ml TE buffer at 60 °C for 10 min. Spin, collect the aqueous phase, and pool it with the saved aqueous phase.

4. Add 0.4 ml of 4 M NaCl and 10 ml of absolute ethanol and chill at −70 °C for 30 min or at −20 °C for 2 h.

5. Centrifuge the tube at 10 000 *g* for 30 min and remove the supernatant by draining the tube on to tissue. Resuspend the pellet in 200 μl of TE buffer, add 100 μl of 7.5 M ammonium acetate, and 600 μl of ethanol. Chill as above, spin for 10 min in a microcentrifuge, dry the pellet under vacuum, and finally resuspend it in 50 μl of TE buffer. Use 10 μl for dot blotting.

B. *For small sections* (13,14)

1. Cut two or three 50 μm sections with a microtome, excise, chop up, and weigh the tissue.

2. Suspend in 0.1 M Tris–HCl buffer pH 8.0 containing 40 mM EDTA, 10 mM NaCl, and 1% SDS, 500 μg/ml of proteinase K. Vortex for 2 min.

Protocol 7. *Continued*

Use less than 10 mg tissue in 0.2 ml of digestion buffer in a 2 ml tube, or 10–30 mg tissue in 1 ml in a 15 ml tube.

3. Incubate at 50 °C for 19 h with constant agitation.

4. Adjust the proteinase K concentration to 1 mg/ml and the SDS concentration to 2% and incubate at 50 °C for 24 h. The proteinase K can be inactivated by heating at 95 °C for 10 min, if necessary.

5. Extract the aqueous phase two or three times with phenol/chloroform/isoamyl alcohol. Add 2 volumes of ethanol, chill, and recover as in steps 4 and 5 of *Protocol 7A*.

[a] The section or block can be dewaxed in a solvent such as xylene before DNA extraction.

There are many commercial kits available for the isolation of DNA or RNA from cells and tissues; however, they are not generally designed for use with clinical and pathological specimens. One popular method involves disruption of the tissue with the chaotropic agent NaI and binding of the DNA to a silica matrix (15). Two kits that we have successfully used following the manufacturer's instructions are those from Bio 101 (the Geneclean kit) and Perkin Elmer (the Isogene kit). The Isogene kit allows the recovery of RNA as well as DNA; however, *Protocol 8* is one of the simplest and direct methods of purifying RNA using silica as the solid phase matrix. For purification of high molecular weight DNA, a diatom suspension (Celite, Janssen Chimica) is used.

Protocol 8. Nucleic acid extraction using silica and guanidinium thiocyanate (16)

Reagents

- Buffer L6: add 120 g of guanidinium thiocyanate[a] (GuSCN; Fluka) to 100 ml of 0.1 M Tris–HCl pH 6.4 and 22 ml of 0.2 M EDTA pH 8.0, and 2.6 g of Triton X-100; stir overnight in the dark to dissolve (buffer L6 is stable for 3 weeks at room temperature in the dark)
- Buffer L2: add 120 g of GuSCN to 100 ml of 0.1 M Tris–HCl pH 6.4; heat with shaking at 60–65 °C to dissolve, or stir overnight in the dark (buffer L2 is stable for 3 weeks at room temperature in the dark)
- Silica: stand 60 g of silicon dioxide (Sigma)

and 500 ml deionized H_2O in a cylinder for 24 h at room temperature. Remove about 430 ml of supernatant, resuspend solids in 500 ml of deionized H_2O. Stand for 5 h at room temperature, remove about 440 ml of supernatant. Add 600 μl of concentrated HCl to pH 2. Aliquot, autoclave, and store in the dark.
- Diatom suspension: for genomic DNA, in place of silica use 10 g of Celite (Janssen Chimica) plus 50 ml of H_2O and 500 μl of concentrated HCl. Aliquot and autoclave.

Method

1. Add 50 μl of specimen to 900 μl of buffer L6 and 40 μl of silica (vortex first) in a Sarstedt screw-capped microfuge tube. The specimen may be

deproteinized by incubation in the presence of 2 mg/ml proteinase K, 0.5% SDS at 37 °C for 30 min before addition to the L6 buffer.

2. Vortex for 5 sec, stand at room temperature for 10 min, vortex for 5 sec, spin for 15 sec in a micro centrifuge, and remove supernatant.

3. Add 1 ml of buffer L2 and vortex, spin for 15 sec, and remove supernatant.

4. Repeat step 3.

5. Repeat step 3 with 70% ethanol, twice.

6. Repeat step 3 with acetone, once.

7. Dry for 10 min at 56 °C with lid open.

8. Add 40–50 μl of TE buffer (*Protocol 4*) or H_2O (plus 1 μl (40 units) of RNase inhibitor, Promega), vortex, incubate at 56 °C for 10 min, vortex, then spin for 2 min at high speed. Addition of proteinase K at 100 ng/ml to the TE buffer may help elution of some DNAs which have bound proteins. However, the proteinase K must subsequently be inactivated (by heating at 95 °C for 10–15 min) if the DNA or RNA is to be reacted with enzymes. If the DNA is to be dot blotted or Southern blotted, inactivation is not necessary.

9. Collect supernatant, taking care not to carry over any silica.[b]

[a] **Caution**: on contact with acids GuSCN can produce HCN. Use fume hood for buffers and collect waste into 10 M NaOH.
[b] Not all of the RNA may be recovered in the first wash, particularly if it is double-stranded RNA. A second and third elution will increase the yield.

Some samples, such as haemolysed blood or faecal specimens, are difficult to use in dot blot hybridization tests since they can block the filter; they are often coloured such that they interfere with a colorimetric detection assay; they can also bind the probe non-specifically. This is a particular problem for faecal samples, which need to be extracted with phenol/chloroform (*Protocol 9*) prior to extraction by *Protocol 8*.

Protocol 9. Extraction of RNA or DNA from faeces

Reagents

• FE medium: 90 ml deionized H_2O, 10 ml 199 medium, 0.1 ml gentamycin, 3.0 ml bicarbonate

• Tris/Ca buffer: 20 mM Tris–HCl pH 8.0, 10 mM NaCl, 3 mM $CaCl_2$

Method

1. Add 0.5 g of solid or 0.2–0.3 ml of liquid faeces to 5 ml of FE medium or Tris/Ca buffer.[a] FE medium is preferable if the faecal extract is also to

Protocol 9. *Continued*

be examined by electron microscopy; Tris/Ca buffer is easier to work with for routine extractions.

2. Vortex and centrifuge at 1500 *g* for 5 min at room temperature.

3. Add 50 μl of 1 M sodium acetate pH 5.0, 1% SDS to 0.45 ml of faecal extract. Mix and add 0.5 ml of 70 % phenol/chloroform mixture (Applied Biosystems). Vortex for 1 min and incubate at 56 °C for 15 min.

4. Microcentrifuge for 2–3 min and remove the upper aqueous phase to a clean microfuge tube. Add 0.1 volume of 3 M sodium acetate and 2 volumes of cold absolute ethanol. Incubate at −70 °C for 30 min or at −20 °C for 2 h to overnight.

5. Microcentrifuge for 10 min. Pour off the supernatant and dry the pellet under vacuum. Resuspend in TE buffer.

6. If the pellet/solution appears 'clean' or colourless it can be applied to a membrane for dot blotting as described in *Protocol 10* or *Protocol 11*. It can also be analysed by gel electrophoresis and Southern/Northern blotting. If the pellet is 'dirty' it can be further cleaned up as described in *Protocol 8*.

---

[a] The use of fluorocarbon solvents (e.g. 'Arcton') to extract the faecal suspension appears to decrease RNA/DNA yield.

3. Blotting

The majority of blotting methods involve denaturation of the nucleic acid and application to a membrane by capillary action under gravity or with suction. Detailed procedures for electrophoresis and for Southern and Northern transfers will not be given here; a molecular biology laboratory manual such as reference 10 should be consulted. Nylon, charged nylon, or strengthened nitrocellulose membranes, available from several suppliers, can all be used. For some colorimetric detection methods nitrocellulose membranes may give a lower background. Standard nylon membranes can be used for routine purposes. The manufacturer's protocols give advice on choosing a membrane for a specific application (e.g. Amersham). Procedures for dot/slot blotting techniques are described in *Protocols 10* and *11*.

There are procedures for 'sandwich' hybridization in which a capture probe complementary to part of the target sequence is bound to the solid phase. The denatured specimen and detector probe (complementary to another region of the target sequence) are added and hybridization occurs between the three sequences (17, 18). Non-hybridized material is washed away and bound probe detected. This technique may give a lower background signal when 'dirty' biological samples are used, but it is probably less sensitive than direct hybridization. However, it is amenable to adaptation to a microtitre plate format.

Protocol 10. DNA dot or slot blotting

1. Combine 10–100 μl of sample (e.g. serum, non-particulate body fluid, or extracted DNA) with 100 μl of denaturing solution (2 M NaCl, 1 M NaOH). Adjust the volume to 200 μl with 10 × SSC (1 × SSC is 0.15 M NaCl, 0.015 M sodium citrate, pH 7.0). Leave at room temperature for 10 min. Urine (100 μl) can be denatured by addition of 25 μl 2.5 M NaCl, 1.5 M NaOH for 30 min at room temperature.

2. Assemble a 'minifold' apparatus (e.g. Schleicher and Schuell) with a pre-wetted (in 10 × SSC) filter paper backing (e.g. Whatman 3MM). Layer on the nylon membrane, smoothing out any air bubbles. Wet the membrane first in deionized H_2O, then in 10 × SSC. Always wear gloves when handling the membrane.

3. Apply the samples to each well with the vacuum running. Once the samples have gone through the membrane, rinse the wells with 200 μl of 10 × SSC or 0.5 M Tris–HCl pH 7.4, 1.5 M NaCl. Carefully disassemble the apparatus and dry the membrane at 37 °C or 80 °C for 2 h. The DNA can be fixed on the membrane by exposure to UV light (e.g. for 2–3 min) according to the manufacturer's instructions.

Protocol 11. RNA dot or slot blotting [a]

1. Incubate the RNA at 65 °C for 5 min in 3 volumes of a solution made up of 500 μl of formamide, 162 μl of 37% formaldehyde, 100 μl of 10 × Mops buffer (0.2 M morpholinopropane-sulphonic acid, 0.05 M sodium acetate, 0.01 M EDTA, pH 7.0). Chill on ice and add an equal volume of 20 × SSC.[a] Alternatively, adjust the RNA solution to 50% deionized formamide/10% formaldehyde buffered with 2 mM phosphate pH 7.0, for 10 min at room temperature, and then add an equal volume of 20 × SSC.

2. Apply to a 'minifold' apparatus as in *Protocol 10*.

[a] Blotting and hybridization protocols, Amersham.

---

4. Production and purification of probes

The probe used in a hybridization experiment is usually from one of four sources:

(a) DNA or RNA purified or transcribed from purified tissue culture grown virus—these type of probes are seldom used nowadays

(b) synthetic oligonucleotide probes which can be bought or made on a commercial machine; they are of limited sensitivity and are best suited for *in situ* hybridization, the detection of PCR products, or the detection of point mutations

(c) DNA or RNA produced from molecular, recombinant clones of virion DNA; these are the most commonly used probes (the cloning of viral genomes is beyond the scope of this chapter—the best sources of cloned genomes are from repositories such as the American Type Culture Collection or colleagues who have already made them)

(d) PCR products can be labelled with ^{32}P or digoxygenin during amplification and used as probes (*Protocol 12*). This approach has the advantage that cloning of the viral genome is not necessary (provided some sequence information is available). Also, after the initial PCR product has been produced and purified away from any non-specifically amplified material, it serves as the template for secondary amplifications. In this way a labelled probe can be produced that is essentially free of any extraneous sequences. This circumvents the main problems associated with the production and use of cloned probes. A cloned probe has to be excised from the vector before it is labelled. Residual, contaminating vector sequences can hybridize with bacterial and phage sequences which sometimes contaminate clinical, pathological, and environmental specimens.

5. Labelling of probes

Radioactive *in vitro* labelling of nucleic acids is described in a companion volume in this series (19). For most applications in clinical virology the choice is between the use of an RNA or a DNA probe. RNA probes are produced by transcription of sequences inserted in a vector with an RNA polymerase promoter (e.g. pSP series or pGEM series). In theory RNA probes offer the advantages of high specific activity, the ability to transcribe only the DNA strand that is complementary to the target virion RNA or DNA, and the greater stability of RNA:RNA and DNA:RNA hybrids over DNA:DNA hybrids. However, in practice, there are difficulties associated with the use of ss RNA probes. Unless the reaction conditions are fully optimized, RNA polymerases can terminate prematurely, producing an excess of short transcripts over the correct full-length product. Also, degradation of ss RNA readily occurs during the processing and hybridization of the RNA probe. Additionally, viral RNAs have sequence homology (particularly in the RNA polymerase/replicase genes) between virus groups and with cellular RNAs. These three effects can combine to give an apparently specific hybridization signal that is difficult to interpret. For this reason I find DNA probes preferable for most dot, slot, and Southern blot experiments.

The viral DNA sequences are cut out from the vector with an appropriate restriction enzyme and purified by agarose gel electrophoresis. There are several methods for achieving this. The use of a Geneclean (Bio 101), Isogene (Perkin Elmer), Qiagen (Diagen) or other commercial kit is recommended.

Radioactive labelling *in vitro* (19) is most conveniently accomplished using a nick translation or random priming kit, available from various manufacturers (Amersham, Pharmacia, Bohringer Mannheim, etc.).

Non-radioactive probes labelled with biotin or digoxygenin can be prepared using kits available from several sources (Life Technologies, Boehringer Mannheim (21), Amersham, etc.).

The use of PCR is described elsewhere in this volume (Chapter 5). The PCR conditions for the sequence to be used as a probe are first established. The PCR is then modified to produce a labelled product. If the PCR uses a fairly crude substrate and non-target bands are visible on gel electrophoresis, the PCR product must be purified before it is used as the substrate of a labelling reaction. This can be accomplished by cutting the correct target band from the gel and recovering it with a Geneclean, Qiagen, or other PCR product purification kit. It is better, however, to optimize the PCR fully so that only the desired band is produced. This can be accomplished by using a high annealing temperature, and short annealing and extension times, thus ensuring that the reaction is as stringent as possible.

Protocol 12. Production of labelled PCR probes

A. *Digoxygenin labelled probes*[a]

1. Combine the following in a 50 μl microcentrifuge tube:
   - 5 μl of 10 × reaction buffer (100 mM Tris–HCl pH 8.3, 500 mM KCl, 15–25 ml MgCl$_2$)
   - 5 μl of 2 mM dATP
   - 5 μl of 2 mM dCTP
   - 5 μl of 2 mM dGTP
   - 3.25 μl of 2 mM TTP
   - 3.5 μl of 1 mM digoxygenin-dUTP[b] (21)
   - 25–50 pmol of each primer
   - 1 ng of template DNA
   - 1.25 units of *Taq* polymerase
   - H$_2$O to 50 μl

Protocol 12. *Continued*

2. Overlay with mineral oil. Cycle 35 times using established conditions.

3. Use the product directly or after purification.

B. *^{32}P-labelled probes* (21)

1. Combine the following in a 50 μl microcentrifuge tube:

   - 5 μl of 10 × reaction buffer (100 mM Tris–HCl pH 8.3, 500 mM KCl, 25 mM MgCl$_2$)
   - 5 μl of 2 mM dATP
   - 5 μl of 2 mM TTP
   - 5 μl of 2 mM dGTP
   - 3 μM [^{32}P]dCTP
   - 25–50 pmol of each primer[c]
   - 1 ng of template DNA
   - 1.25 units of *Taq* polymerase
   - H$_2$O to 50 μl

2. Overlay with mineral oil. Cycle 35 times using established conditions.

3. Use the product directly or after purification.

---

[a] Biotinylated probes can also be produced using biotin-dUTP and TTP in a ratio of 1:3. In preliminary experiments 'Vent' DNA polymerase (New England Biolabs) was observed to perform better with biotin-dUTP than *Taq* polymerase.
[b] This is a ratio of 6.5:3.5 of TTP to digoxygenin-dUTP.
[c] Strand-specific DNA probes can be produced by asymmetric PCR (22).

Oligonucleotides can be labelled at the 5'-end using polynucleotide kinase and [γ-^{32}P]ATP (19), by priming with a complementary oligonucleotide using Klenow fragment in the presence of [^{32}P]dNTP (23), or at the 3'-end using terminal transferase (see *Protocol 13* and reference 24). If oligonucleotides are labelled at the 5'-end they can be extended by DNA polymerases which require a 3'-OH group to initiate DNA synthesis. This property is exploited in some DNA sequencing and PCR protocols and also as a method to detect PCR products (25). The main disadvantage of labelling the 5'-end is that polynucleotide kinase preferentially labels short oligonucleotides, thus it is essential that the synthetic DNA probe is pure.

Terminal transferase can be used to add either a 'tail' of labelled bases at the 3'-end, or just one base if a chain terminator is used in the reaction. Although most tailed oligonucleotides work in practice, there may be situations where the tail of non-homologous nucleotides disrupts the stability of the probe under stringent hybridization and washing conditions.

Protocol 13. 3′-end labelling of oligonucleotides

1. Combine the following in this order:

- 15 μl of H_2O
- 1 μl of oligonucleotide (50–100 pmol)
- 12.5 μl of 280 mM cacodylic acid, adjusted to pH 7.0 with KOH, 0.56 mM dithiothreitol
- 2.5 μl of 14 mM $CoCl_2$
- 3.0 μl of [^{32}P]dATP (3000–5000 Ci/mmol)[a]
- 1.0 μl of terminal transferase (Amersham; 5–10 units)

2. Incubate at 37 °C for 30 min.

3. Purify the oligonucleotide either by gel filtration on Sephadex G-50 (e.g. using a Pharmacia 'Nick' column) or by ethanol precipitation as follows. Adjust the volume to 200 μl by adding 20 μl of 10% SDS, 100 μg of nuclease-free glycogen (Boehringer Mannheim), and H_2O. Add 100 μl of 7.5 M ammonium acetate and 900 μl of absolute ethanol. Mix and chill at −70 °C for 30 min, then pellet in a microcentrifuge for 15–30 min.

4. Determine the counts incorporated by a DEAE binding assay (19). There should be a total of at least 10^7 c.p.m.

[a] Digoxygenin-dUTP (100 μM) can also be incorporated (20).

---

6. Hybridization and detection

After the DNA/RNA has been fixed, the membrane is put in a plastic bag or hybridization oven tube for hybridization (10). Commonly, hybridization is at 68°C in aqueous solution (*Protocol 14*), at 42°C in formamide (*Protocol 15*), or *in situ* (*Protocol 16*). A hybridization protocol for characterization of PCR products is provided in Chapter 5.

Protocol 14. Hybridization in aqueous solution[a]

Reagents

- Hybridization solution: 30 ml 20 × SSC, 5 ml 10% SDS, 5 ml 0.2 M EDTA pH 7.4, 2 ml of 5 × Denhardt's solution, 100 μg/ml denatured salmon sperm DNA, H_2O to 100 ml
- 2 × SSC (see *Protocol 10*), 0.1% SDS
- 1 × SSC, 0.1% SDS
- 0.2 × SSC, 0.1% SDS
- 5 mM Tris–HCl pH 8.0, 2 mM EDTA *or* 0.4 m NaOH
- Neutralization solution: 0.2 M Tris–HCl pH 7.4, 0.1 × SSC, 0.1% SDS

Method

1. Warm hybridization solution to 68 °C.

2. Add just enough hybridization solution to keep the filter moist and

Protocol 14. *Continued*

incubate at 68 °C for 30 min (either submerged in a water bath or hybridization oven).

3. Denature the probe by heating at 95–100 °C for 5–10 min in hybridization solution. Add it to the membrane and continue incubation for 4–16 h.

4. Remove the membrane to 2 × SSC, 0.1% SDS and wash off excess hybridization solution at room temperature.

5. Wash the membrane at 68 °C progressively, for 15 min each on a shaker, in: 2 × SSC, 0.1% SDS; 1 × SSC, 0.1% SDS; 0.2 × SSC, 0.1% SDS.

6. Blot the membrane dry (but do not allow it to dry completely if it is to be re-probed) and develop it colorimetrically or seal it in a plastic bag and expose it to X-ray film.

7. Specifically bound ^{32}P-labelled probe can be removed and the blot re-probed by washing it in either 5 mM Tris–HCl pH 8.0, 2 mM EDTA for 2 h at 68 °C or 0.4 M NaOH at 4 °C for 30 min, followed by neutralization in neutralization solution for 15 min (Amersham protocols). The membrane should be re-exposed to X-ray film to check that all probe has been removed before re-hybridization

[a] This is used with nick-translated or random primed probes.

Protocol 15. Hybridization in formamide solutions [a]

Reagents

- Hybridization solution: 30 ml of 20 × SSC, 5 ml of 10% SDS, 0.4 ml of 5% Denhardt's solution, 30 ml of deionized formamide pH 7.0, H₂O to 100 ml [b]
- 2 × SSC (see *Protocol 10*), 0.1% SDS

- 3.0 m tetramethylammonium chloride, 50 mM Tris–HCl pH 7.0, 2 mM EDTA, 0.1% SDS
- 5 mM Tris–HCl pH 8.0, 2 mM EDTA

Method

1. Warm hybridization solution to 42 °C.

2. Add just enough solution to keep the membrane moist and incubate at 42 °C for 30 min (either submerged in a water bath or in a hybridization oven).

3. Add the labelled probe to the membrane and continue incubation for 4–16 h.

4. Remove the membrane to 2 × SSC, 0.1% SDS and wash off the excess hybridization solution at room temperature.

5. Wash the membrane in the above solution at 42 °C for 2 h, blot it dry (but do not allow it to dry completely if it is to be re-probed), and develop it colorimetrically or seal it in a plastic bag and expose it to X-ray film.

6. Alternatively, the membrane can be washed in 3.0 M tetramethyl-ammonium chloride, 50 mM Tris–HCl pH 7.0, 2 mM EDTA, 0.1% SDS at 60 °C.

7. Specifically bound ^{32}P-labelled probe can be removed and the blot re-probed by washing it in 5 mM Tris–HCl pH 8.0, 2 mM EDTA for 2 h at 68 °C (Amersham protocols). The membrane should be re-exposed to X-ray film to check all probe has been removed before re-hybridization

[a] Used for hybridization with oligonucleotide probes.
[b] Carrier DNA is not used for hybridization with short oligonucleotides; it may bind the probe.

Protocol 16. *In situ* hybridization (26)

Reagents

- Hybridization solution: 45% deionized formamide pH 6.8, 5 × SSC, 2.5% polyethylene glycol, 800 μg/ml carrier DNA, 3 μg/ml probe DNA
- 3-Aminopropyltriethyl oxysilane (Sigma)
- Carnoy's fluid (75 ml ethanol, 25 ml glacial acetic acid)
- Ethanol (100%, and 70 and 50% in H_2O)
- Xylene

- Proteinase K (10–500 μg/ml in 50 mM Tris–HCl pH 7.5, 100 mM KCl, 5 mM mgCl)
- 4 × SSC (see *Protocol 10*)
- PBS
- 0.1% Triton X-100 m PBS
- PBS containing 5 mM EDTA, 0.5% Triton X-100, 0.1% BSA
- 0.3 m ammonium acetate in 70% ethanol and 90% ethanol

Method

1. Treat slides with 3-aminopropyltriethyloxysilane. Fix 5 μM sections of unfixed tissue on them for 10 min in Carnoy's fluid. Formaldehyde-fixed, paraffin-embedded sections (5 μm) are placed on similarly treated slides and baked at 60 °C for 30 min. They are dewaxed in xylene for 5 min, then taken through a graded series of ethanols (100%, and 70% and 50% in H_2O, for 2 min each) and treated with proteinase K (10–500 μg/ml in 50 mM Tris–HCl pH 7.5, 100 mM KCl, 5 mM $MgCl_2$, at 55 °C for 2 h to overnight, depending on the resistance of the tissue).

2. Add 5–30 μl of hybridization solution, depending on the size of the coverslip, and seal with gum (e.g. 'Cow gum' diluted 1:1 with ether). Dry for 10 min at room temperature.

3. Bake at 90 °C for 10 min to denature the probe and specimen DNA and hybridize at 37 °C overnight in a moist chamber.

4. Remove the coverslips under 4 × SSC, wash three times in 4 × SSC,

Protocol 16. *Continued*

once with 0.1% Triton X-100 in PBS, and once with PBS (each wash for 5 min at room temperature).

5. Develop the signal depending on whether the probe is non-radioactive or radioactive. For example, a non-radioactive detection complex is diluted 1:200 in PBS, containing 5 mM EDTA, 0.5% Triton X-100, 0.1% BSA and incubated at room temperature for 30 min, and then processed according to the manufacturer's instructions. If the probe is radioactive ([3]H- or ^{35}S-labelled) the slides are dehydrated in 0.3 M ammonium acetate in 70% ethanol after the 4 × SSC washes, then in 0.3 M ammonium acetate in 90% ethanol. Dry the slides at room temperature, dip in Ilford G5 nuclear emulsion, expose, and develop in Kodak D19 developer and rapid fixer.

7. Example: parvovirus B19 DNA

An example of detection of viral nucleic acid by dot hybridization is given in *Protocol 17* for parvovirus B19 DNA.

Protocol 17. Dot hybridization detection of parvovirus B19 DNA

A. *Application of specimens to membrane*

1. To each well of a microtitre plate add 90 μl of 2 × SSC (see *Protocol 10*) and 100 μl of 2 M NaCl, 1 M NaOH.

2. Add 10 μl of sample (e.g. serum or plasma) or control (e.g. known positive B19 serum or cloned B19 DNA[a]) to each well and allow about 15 min for denaturation at room temperature.

3. Identify membrane (e.g. positively charged nylon membrane from Boehringer Mannheim) by marking in pencil in the top left hand corner.

4. Equilibrate membrane and blotting paper (Schleicher and Schuell or Whatman 3 MM) in 2 × SSC. Assemble blotting paper and membrane in a 'minifold' apparatus. Make sure no air bubbles are trapped.

5. Transfer the whole contents of the wells of the microtitre plate to the corresponding wells of the minifold apparatus. Apply vacuum for a few minutes until all of the solution has passed through the membrane.

6. Remove the membrane and rinse briefly in 2 × SSC. Place the membrane between 3 MM paper and dry at 120 °C for 20 min.

B. *DNA labelling with biotin or digoxygenin*

1. Prepare cloned B19 DNA excised from the plasmid vector and re-covered by gel electrophoresis and the use of a 'Geneclean' kit.

2. Label the DNA using either a biotin nick translation kit from Life Technologies or a digoxygenin DNA labelling kit from Boehringer Mannheim, or another suitable kit (see *Protocol 12*).

3. Purify the probe using either a Sephadex G-50 column under gravity, or a spun column, or ethanol precipitation from 3.75 M ammonium acetate.

C. *Hybridization, and chemiluminescent and colorimetric detection* (*Protocol 13*)

1. Soak membrane in 2 × SSC until uniformly hydrated. Seal in a plastic bag (two membranes may be placed back to back) with 20 ml of hybridization solution (5 × SSC, 2% blocking reagent (Boehringer Mannheim), 0.1% *n*-laurylsarcosine, 0.02% SDS). Incubate at 68°C for at least 1 h in a shaking water bath.

2. Denature the probe by heating at 95–100°C for 10 min, and snap-cool on ice. Add to 10 ml of hybridization solution, and replace the pre-hybridization solution. Incubate for a further 16 h at 68°C in a shaking water bath.

3. Remove the hybridization solution.[b]

4. Wash at room temperature for 2 × 5 min in 100 ml per membrane of 2 × SSC, 0.1% SDS.

5. Wash at 68°C for 2 × 5 min in 100 ml per membrane of 0.1 × SSC, 0.1% SDS.

6. If the probe is labelled with biotin, develop the membrane according to the manufacturer's instructions (e.g. Life Technologies). If the membrane is dried before colour development it must be rehydrated before use. Nitrocellulose membranes give a lower background than nylon membranes; however, they cannot be re-used because the dyes used in the colour development appear to bind irreversibly to the membrane. The dyes can be removed from nylon membranes (see *Protocol 14*).

7. If the probe is labelled with digoxygenin it can be first developed using an anti-digoxygenin–alkaline phosphatase conjugate and AMPDD (3-(2′-spiroadamantane)-4-methoxy-4-(3′-phosphoryloxy)-phenyl-1,2-dioxetane; Boehringer Mannheim), then sealed, while still damp, in a plastic bag and exposed to X-ray film (e.g. Hyperfilm-MP, Amersham) for 10 min to 1 h. AMPDD is a chemiluminescent substrate for alkaline phosphatase.

8. To follow chemiluminescence with colour detection, wash membranes briefly in 100 mM Tris–HCl pH 9.5, 100 mM NaCl, 50 mM $MgCl_2$, then

Protocol 17. *Continued*

proceed directly to colour detection by adding NBT/BCIP solution (4-nitro blue tetrazolium chloride and 5-bromo-4-chloro-3-indolyl-phosphate; Boehringer Mannheim). After stopping the colour development, dry the membrane and seal in a plastic bag for permanent storage.

[a] A dilution series of either or both of these positive controls is advisable.
[b] The hybridization solution should be recovered and stored at −20 °C for further use. For re-use it should be transferred to a Corex tube, denatured in a boiling water bath for 10 min, and snap-cooled on ice.

8. Trouble shooting

Loss or degradation of DNA, and particularly RNA, during transport and processing of specimens is one of the main problems of using nucleic detection as a means of diagnosing viral infections. This can be overcome by keeping specimens cold or frozen during transport to the laboratory, and by the use of RNase inhibitors in transport media. Once in the laboratory the specimens should be kept frozen, preferably at −70 °C, or processed immediately. Solutions should be filtered through 0.45 μM membranes and autoclaved where possible. Additionally, solutions for RNA work should be treated with DEPC and free of divalent cations such as Mn^{2+}. Gloves should be worn when preparing intact RNA, and pipettes and apparatus should be sterile (autoclaved) and dedicated to RNA work, and never be used with nucleases.

High backgrounds on X-ray film when ^{32}P-labelled probes are used are usually due to incomplete removal of unincorporated labelled nucleotides. Problems are also caused by the presence of air bubbles in the hybridization solution, incomplete wetting of the membrane, or membranes touching during hybridization and washing. A second round of washing may solve this problem. If not, strip the membrane (*Protocol 14*) and re-probe.

The interpretation of the results of colorimetric non-radioactive detection systems can be problematic if the specimen itself is coloured. Some biological materials contain endogenous biotin which can result in false positives if a biotin labelling system is used (7). For these reasons a digoxygenin-labelled probe is preferable.

When probes derived from sequences cloned in bacterial vectors are used, residual vector sequences may cross-hybridize with bacteria contaminating the clinical specimen (7,27–29). If there is sufficient viral DNA present in the specimen it may be possible to separate the target DNA and the contaminating DNA by electrophoresis, and to determine the size of the hybridizing sequences by Southern blotting and hybridization. Alternatively, an excess of the vector DNA can be included in the hybridization solution to compete out any labelled residual vector DNA. The pre-hybridization solution should still contain a non-homologous blocking agent such as salmon or herring sperm DNA. These problems should not arise if synthetic oligonucleotides or PCR products are used as probes.

9. Significance of viral nucleic acid detection

Detection of viral nucleic acid has found its place when viruses cannot be grown easily or at all and when nucleic acid detection is an important complement to serological techniques (e.g. for hepatitis B and C viruses, human papillomaviruses, human parvoviruses, and HIV).

It is obviously a truism that viral RNA or DNA can only be detected if the virus itself is present. After initial infection most viruses produce a viraemia that lasts until it is counter-acted by the host's immune response. After this, the virus is either cleared, leaving the host with some degree of immunity to further infection, or it establishes a persistent or latent infection with low or no viraemia, respectively. Dot blot or Southern hybridization is only sufficiently sensitive to detect the initial (intense) viraemia for some viruses, for instance B19 and hepatitis B viruses. The viraemia of other viruses, particularly RNA viruses (e.g. HIV, picornaviruses, and influenza viruses) needs to be sought by amplification techniques such as PCR. This is partly because these viruses produce nucleic acid only in a few tissues, and partly because serum is often not an appropriate specimen for laboratory analysis. Those specimens that are more appropriate (faeces or throat swabs for picornaviruses and influenzaviruses, respectively) are not conducive for the survival of RNA in an easily detectable form. Although by no means always the case, it may be that by the time the patient presents with symptoms, the levels of virus are declining (e.g. B19).

Serological tests (rising or declining antibody titres, specific IgM; antigen detection, etc.) are common diagnostic tests in a microbiological laboratory. Application of DNA or RNA detection needs to be carefully targeted. It is important to consider whether, and in what form, viral nucleic acid is likely to be present in any specimen to be analysed:

(a) Does the virus replicate in, or spread to this specimen?

(b) Is it still present when symptoms develop?

(c) Is the genome likely to survive transport in a necrotic tissue, full of nucleases?

(d) If present, is it likely to be at a sufficiently high titre to be detectable by direct hybridization, or is PCR necessary?

(e) If PCR is to be used, have the samples been handled correctly to avoid contamination, and are there sufficient controls (e.g. at the time of collection of the sample) for any result to be meaningful and interpretable?

If the viral sequences are detectable by PCR alone, what is the significance of a low level of infection? Does it imply a resolving acute infection (e.g. B19); or asymptomatic carriage; or latency (e.g. cytomegalovirus or HBV), or does it suggest changes in the status of a chronic infection, for example in response to drug therapy (e.g. HBV), or a relapsing or recurring infection at the end of a therapeutic regime (e.g. B19, HCV)?

(f) Is the virus likely to be latent or persistent and, if so, is it more appropriate to search for mRNA than virion RNA or DNA?

(g) Will the probe (or primers) detect all members of the virus (quasi) species (e.g. HIV)?

(h) Will it be necessary to sequence any detected DNA/RNA to characterize it definitively?

(i) Will the probe (or primers) cross-hybridize with cellular genes, endogenous viral sequences, or contaminating bacteria?

(j) Can a DNA/RNA hybridization result be confirmed by another independent technique?

Acknowledgements

Many thanks to colleagues who contributed and tested protocols: Mark Broughton, Bernard Cohen, Chris Gallimore, Kate Gibson, Pat Gibson, Nick Hallam, Julie Mori, Jussara Nascimento, and Andrea Thomas.

References

1. Winn-Deen, E. S., Batt, C. A., and Wiedmann, M. (1993). *Mol. Cell Probes*, **7**, 179.
2. Fahrlander, P. D. (1988). *Biotechnology*, **6**, 1165.
3. Mize, P. D., Hoke, R. A., Linn, C. P., Reardon, J. E., and Schulte, T. H. (1989). *Anal. Biochem.*, **179**, 229.
4. Meinkoth, J. and Wahl, G. (1984). *Anal. Biochem.*, **138**, 267.
5. Hames, B. D. and Higgins, S. J. (eds) (1985). *Nucleic acid hybridization, a practical approach*. IRL Press, Oxford, UK.
6. Keller, G. H. and Manak, M. M. (1989). *DNA Probes*. Stockton Press, New York.
7. Mori, J., Field, A. M., Clewley, J. P., and Cohen, B. J. (1989). *J. Clin. Microbiol.*, **27**, 459.
8. Jackson, J. B. (1991). *Am. J. Clin. Pathol.*, **95**, 442.
9. Roman, A. and Fife, K. H. (1989). *Clin. Microbiol. Rev.*, **2**, 166.
10. Sambrook, J., Fritsch, E. F., and Maniatis, T. (1989). *Molecular cloning, a laboratory manual*, 2nd edn. Cold Spring Harbor Laboratory Press, Cold Spring Harbor, NY.
11. Gibson, K. M., McLean, K. A., and Clewley, J. P. (1991). *J. Virol. Methods*, **32**, 277.

12. Hirt, B. (1967). *J. Mol. Biol.*, **26**, 365.
13. Goelz, S. E., Hamilton, S. R., and Vogelstein, B. (1985). *Biochem. Biophys. Res. Commun.*, **120**, 118.
14. Imprain, C. C., Saiki, R. K., Erlich, H. A., and Teplitz, R. L. (1987). *Biochem. Biophys. Res. Commun.*, **142**, 710.
15. Vogelstein, B. and Gillespie, D. (1979). *Proc. Natl. Acad. Sci. USA*, **76**, 615.
16. Boom, R., Sol, C. J. A., Salimans, M. M. M., Lansen, C. L., Wertheim-van Dillen, P. M. E., and van der Noordaa, J. (1990). *J. Clin. Microbiol.*, **28**, 495.
17. Wolf, H., Leser, U., Haus, M., Gu, S. Y., and Pathmanathan, R. (1986). *J. Virol. Methods*, **13**, 1.
18. Nakagami, S., Matsunaga, H., Miyoshi, K., and Yamane, A. (1991). *Anal. Biochem.*, **192**, 11.
19. Cunningham, M. W., Harris, D. W., and Mundy, C. R. (1990). In *Radioisotopes in biology, a practical approach* (ed. R. J. Slater), pp. 137–91. IRL Press, Oxford.
20. Anonymous (1989). *Dig DNA labelling and detection, applications manual.* Boehringer Mannheim, Germany.
21. Jansen, R. and Ledley, F. D. (1989). *Gene Anal. Techn.*, **6**, 79.
22. Sturzl, M. and Roth, W. K. (1990). *Anal. Biochem.*, **185**, 164.
23. Saluz, H. and Jost, J. P. (1989). *Proc. Natl. Acad. Sci. USA.*, **86**, 2602.
24. Yousaf, S. I., Carroll, A. R., and Clarke, B. E. (1984). *Gene*, **27**, 309.
25. Parker, J. D. and Burmer, G. C. (1991). *Biotechniques*, **10**, 94.
26. Nascimento, J. P., Hallam, N. F., Mori, J., Field, A. M., Clewley, J. P., Brown, K. E., and Cohen, B. J. (1991). *J. Med. Virol.*, **33**, 77.
27. Ambinder, R. F., Charache, P., Staal, S., Wright, P., Forman, M., Hayward, D., and Hayward, G. S. (1986). *J. Clin. Microbiol.*, **24**, 16.
28. Howell, M. D. and Kaplan, N. O. (1987). *Anal. Biochem.*, **161**, 311.
29. Tabrizi, S. N., Borg, A. J., and Garland, M. (1991). *J. Virol. Methods*, **32**, 41.

4

Blotting of viral proteins

SALLY E. ADAMS and NIGEL R. BURNS

1. Introduction

Blotting techniques are widely applied for assessing the binding of specific antibodies to viral antigens. Such procedures can be used to characterize either the antigen or the antibody. The spectrum of the humoral response against different viral proteins following infection can be determined by using defined antigen preparations. Conversely, defined antibody preparations, of either clinical or experimental origin, can be used to detect the presence of viral antigens in clinical specimens. The application of blotting techniques in medical virology has increased in importance over the last five years with the introduction of confirmatory Western blot assays for the detection of human pathogens such as human immunodeficiency virus (HIV; references 1 and 2), human T cell leukaemia virus type I (HTLV-I; reference 3), and hepatitis C virus (HCV; reference 4). In addition, the scope of blotting procedures has widened with the development of rapid dot and slot blotting methods utilizing recombinant proteins and peptides (5–7), thereby facilitating detailed analysis of the immune response elicited by a particular virus and giving further insight into disease progression and pathogenesis.

The process of blotting viral proteins can be broadly divided into two components. Firstly, a source of viral protein needs to be identified and the antigen prepared for analysis. Secondly, the viral protein is blotted on to a suitable support matrix followed by probing with antibody and detection of bound reagents. The purpose of this chapter is to outline general methods for preparing viral antigens for blotting, to describe various procedures for blotting proteins and detecting bound antibodies, and to assess the advantages and disadvantages of these alternatives.

2. Isolation of viral proteins

2.1 Sources of viral proteins

Viral proteins required for blotting purposes may be obtained from *ex vivo* samples, tissue culture grown material, or recombinant micro-organisms expressing specific viral antigens. In some instances it may be preferable to use short synthetic peptides in blotting procedures in order to determine the binding specificity of a particular antibody.

2.2 Laboratory safety

Safety is an important issue in all laboratories, but is of particular priority in laboratories dealing with human pathogens and clinical samples. Before commencing work with potential pathogens reference should be made to the guidelines of the Advisory Committee on Dangerous Pathogens entitled *Categorisation of pathogens according to hazard and categories of containment* or other equivalent national guidelines.

2.3 Inactivation procedures

In certain circumstances it may be necessary to inactivate the virus prior to preparation for blotting. The procedure required will obviously depend on the virus to be inactivated. Furthermore, it should be noted that inactivation of the virus may result in the destruction of particular epitopes. As an example, a procedure for inactivation of HIV using β-propiolactone (BPL) is given in *Protocol 1*.

Protocol 1. Inactivation using β-propiolactone (BPL)

A. *Antigen inactivation*[a]

1. Add BPL[b] (Sigma) to 1 ml of cell lysate to give a final concentration of 0.25%.
2. Add three drops of phenol red (0.5% (w/v) solution).
3. Incubate at 4°C for 2 h. Monitor the pH by noting the colour of the indicator dye and restore red coloration if necessary every 15 min using 0.1 M sodium hydroxide.
4. Transfer to 37°C and incubate for 30 min. Monitor the pH and restore red coloration every 15 min using 0.1 M sodium hydroxide.
5. Prepare aliquots of the material and store at −20°C or −89°C.[c]

B. *Serum inactivation*[a]

1. Add BPL to the serum or plasma sample to give a final concentration of 0.25%.
2. Incubate for 1 h at room temperature.
3. Prepare aliquots of the material and store at −20°C or −80°C.[c]

[a] These procedures must be carried out in accordance with adequate safety controls (see Section 2.2).
[b] BPL is a potential carcinogen and must be handled accordingly. Cans must be opened inside a microbiological safety cabinet or fume hood. Fresh BPL should be used for each inactivation.
[c] The inactivation procedure should be validated prior to further handling of the material by testing for loss of infectivity using suitable susceptible cells.

2.4 *Ex vivo* material

In most instances of viral infections tissue biopsies are not required for detecting the presence of viral antigens. Most diseases are sufficiently characteristic that the presence of virus in secretions, blood, or cerebrospinal fluid can provide direct evidence for infection of particular organs. However, in certain cases, for example encephalitis caused by herpes simplex virus, virus can only be found by biopsy of the involved tissue. As these instances are rare, we will not discuss biopsy specimens further but recommend that the investigator follow specific procedures available in the literature (8).

It is unusual for clinical fluids to be analysed directly for the presence of proteins by blotting procedures due to a combination of low levels of viral antigens present and the existence of many highly sensitive and quantitative antigen capture assays, usually in an enzyme-linked immunosorbent assay (ELISA) format. Again, there are exceptions to this and in some infections it may be possible to find high levels of viral proteins, for example in the fluid from vesicles containing herpes simplex virus. In these cases, the sample can be prepared for gel electrophoresis as described in *Protocol 5*.

In order to carry out blotting analyses of clinical specimens, the most common procedure is to increase the amount of virus by co-cultivating cells from infected samples with susceptible cells *in vitro*. Details of some tissue culture techniques for growing viruses from clinical samples are described in Chapter 1 and will not be discussed further here. The procedures for preparing antigen from these cultures are described in the following section.

2.5 Tissue culture derived material

Viral proteins can be derived from either the cells or supernatants of infected tissue cultures.

2.5.1 Cell lysate preparation

There are many buffers and detergents that have been used to produce cell lysates. However, a major problem is often the presence of high molecular weight nucleic acids which results in a thick, viscous solution. This can be overcome by shearing the nucleic acid through a needle, although this is inadvisable if the cells are infected with a human pathogen. *Protocol 2* describes the preparation of a cell lysate using a buffer which does not usually produce a viscous solution.

Protocol 2. Cell lysate preparation

Reagents

- Lysis buffer: 3% (w/v) SDS, 5% (v/v) β-mercaptoethanol, 10% (v/v) glycerol, 6 M urea, 60 mM Tris pH 6.8.
- PBS: dissolve 8.0 g of NaCl, 0.2 g of KCl, 1.44 g of Na_2HPO_4 and 0.24 g of KH_2PO_4 in 800 ml of distilled water. Adjust the pH to 7.2 and make up to 1 litre.

Protocol 2. *Continued*

Method[a]

1. Count the cells and determine cell concentration.

2. Pellet the cells by centrifugation.

3. Wash the pellet in PBS.

4. Resuspend the pellet in lysis buffer, using 10^7 cells per 100 μl of buffer.[b]

5. Heat the sample at 100 °C in an oil bath for 10 min.

6. Centrifuge the sample at 13 500 *g* for 5 min.

7. Discard the pellet and store the supernatant in aliquots at −20 °C.

---

[a] These procedures must be carried out in accordance with adequate safety controls (see Section 2.2).

[b] The ratio of cells to buffer given is suitable for analysis of HIV proteins from infected human T-cell lines. However, it may be necessary to adjust this for other virus/cell combinations.

2.5.2 Concentration of virus from cell supernatants

There are numerous methods described in the literature for concentrating and/or purifying viruses, and the method of choice is largely dependent on the virus involved. A review of virus purification procedures is beyond the scope of this chapter and the reader is referred to general virology texts (for example, reference 9) as a starting point for identifying procedures for specific viruses.

2.6 Recombinant proteins

Many laboratories now use recombinant viral proteins as a source of antigen for blotting purposes. Recombinant sources of antigen are particularly useful where a genetically defined reagent is required for analysis of an uncharacterized polyclonal antiserum or to confirm reactivity of a monoclonal antibody with a specific viral protein. Many systems are available for high level expression of gene products in a range of host cells (reviewed in reference 10). In order to produce antigen for use in blotting procedures it is not normally necessary to purify the recombinant protein. Our discussion of preparing recombinant viral proteins will therefore be limited to describing procedures used to produce lysates from different expression systems.

2.6.1 Lysates derived from *Escherichia coli*

Various methods have been described for enzymatic and mechanical lysis of bacteria containing recombinant proteins. *Protocol 3* describes a method for lysing bacteria with egg white lysozyme followed by sonication to disrupt the viscous lysate. Alternative lysis methods include mechanical agitation with abrasives such as glass beads and liquid shear lysis using a French press (11). If a sonicator is not available, nucleic acids can be removed by treatment with RNases and DNase. A particularly useful enzyme is Benzonase (Boehringer) which is an endonuclease derived from *Serratia marcescens* that degrades both DNA and RNA.

Protocol 3. Preparation of lysates derived from *Escherichia coli*

Reagents

- Lysis buffer: 50 mM Tris–HCl pH 8.0, 50 mM NaCl, 1 mM EDTA, 0.1 mM phenyl-methylsulphonyl fluoride (PMSF)[a]
- 20 mg/ml solution of hen egg lysozyme,

made fresh just before the solution is required
- 5% (v/v) deoxycholate
- 5 × sample buffer: see *Protocol 5*

Method

1. Grow cells to an OD (at 600 nm) of 1.0–1.3. Harvest the cells by centrifugation at 5 000 *g* for 5 min and resuspend the pellet in 20 ml of lysis buffer.[b]

2. Add 200 μl of lysozyme solution. Mix well and stand on ice for 20 min.

3. Add 840 μl of deoxycholate. Mix well and stand on ice for 20 min.

4. Sonicate the mixture for three 15 sec bursts using a sonicator (Fred Baker Scientific). Cool the sonicate on ice between pulses. After sonication, the solution should no longer be viscous.

5. Add 5.25 ml of 5× sample buffer. Mix well.

6. Boil the mixture for 5 min. Cool on ice.

7. Centrifuge the mixture at 15 000 *g* for 30 min to pellet the debris.

8. Transfer supernatant to a fresh tube and store at −2 °C in aliquots.

[a] PMSF must be handled with care. Stock solutions are made in ethanol and should be prepared fresh as required.
[b] This procedure can be scaled down as required.

2.6.2 Yeast cell-derived lysates

Saccharomyces cerevisiae is the yeast most commonly used for expression studies. A wide range of *E. coli*/yeast shuttle vectors has been developed (reviewed in reference 10). The choice of yeast strain to use for expression studies can be important if the protein of interest is susceptible to proteolytic degradation. In particular, it is advisable to use strains which are deficient in major yeast proteases such as carboxypeptidase Y, protease A, and protease B (10). As with *E. coli*, either enzymatic or mechanical breakage can be employed to produce yeast cell lysates. However, the impurity of some enzymatic preparations can result in proteolysis and mechanical methods are therefore often preferred. *Protocol 4* describes mechanical breakage of yeast cells, on a small scale, using glass beads. Large-scale mechanical breakage can be achieved using mechanical bead mills, French presses, or homogenizers (11).

Protocol 4. Preparation of yeast cell lysates

Equipment and reagents

- Sterile, acid-washed 40-mesh glass beads (Sigma)[a]
- TEN buffer: 140 mM NaCl, 1 mM EDTA,
- 10 mM Tris–HCl pH 7.4, containing 01 mM PMSF[b]
- 5 × sample buffer: see *Protocol 5*

Method

1. Resuspend 2–4 × $10-10^{10}$ cells in a Falcon tube in 10 ml of TEN buffer containing containing 0.1 mM PMSF.

2. Centrifuge at 5000 *g* for 5 min to pellet cells.

3. Discard the supernatant.

4. Resuspend pellet in 4 ml of TEN buffer containing 0.1 mM PMSF and add 5 *g* of sterile glass beads.

5. Ensure that the top of the Falcon tube is secured tightly and vortex vigorously for 5 min.

6. Centrifuge at 5000 g for 5 min.

7. Remove the supernatant and keep cold on ice.

8. Repeat steps 4–6 and pool the supernatants.

9. Add 1/4 volume of 5 × sample buffer.

10. Boil the sample for 3 min.

11. Centrifuge at 5000 g for 5 min.

12. Discard the pellet and store the supernatant in aliquots at − 20 °C.

---

[a] Wash the glass beads in concentrated sulphuric acid, rinse 10 times with tap water and twice with distilled water, and dry in a hot air oven. Sterilize the beads by baking at 200 °C for 2 h. Take appropriate precautions when handling concentrated sulphuric acid (for example, wear a full face mask and use acid in a fume hood).

[b] PMSF must be handled with care. Stock solutions are made in ethanol and should be prepared fresh as required.

2.6.3 Lysates of insect and mammalian cells

The expression of heterologous proteins in insect cells using recombinant baculoviruses or in mammalian cells is becoming increasingly popular. Basic protocols for expressing proteins in insect cells have been described by Lukow and Summers (12), and techniques for expressing proteins in mammalian cells have been reviewed by Goeddel (10). Mammalian and insect cell expression systems can be particularly useful for expressing viral glycoproteins. However, glycosylation is not necessarily an advantage when the protein is analysed by blotting following SDS–polyacrylamide gel electrophoresis, since the presence of different glycosylation forms (and hence, different molecular weights) leads to smearing of bands on the gel.

Cell extracts can be prepared from both insect and mammalian cells by simple lysis as described in *Protocol 2*.

3. Blotting

With the exception of protein sequencing studies, all protein or peptide blotting methods comprise three distinct phases:

(a) transfer of the protein or peptide to a suitable matrix (membrane)

(b) probing the matrix with specific antibody

(c) detection of the antibody probe

In the case of Western blotting (13,14), proteins or peptides are electrophoretically transferred to the membrane following gel electrophoresis (see *Figure 1*), whereas dot or slot blotting techniques involve direct application of the proteins or peptides on to the membrane. Western blotting has the advantage that it encompasses a high resolution separation step (gel electrophoresis) from which information, such as the relative molecular mass (M_r) of the target protein, can be determined. Most gel electrophoresis systems involve the denaturing of the protein. Therefore some antigenic sites may be lost. This is not usually a problem if polyclonal antibodies are being used to probe the blot, but may be a problem if a monoclonal antibody is to be applied. Dot and slot blotting (6,7) are quicker than Western blotting and are

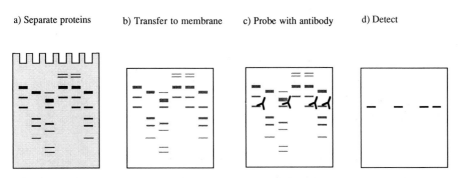

Figure 1. Schematic diagram of steps of Western blotting. Cell lysates or peptides are electrophoretically separated (a; *Protocol 5*), transferred on to a membrane (b; *Protocols 6 and 7*), and probed with specific antibody (c) which in turn is then detected (d; *Protocols 8 and 9*).

particularly suited for a high throughput of samples. Although slot blotting cannot be used to determine the size distribution of the target species, this method is very amenable to quantitative analysis of the response.

3.1 Choice of blotting matrix

Nitrocellulose membranes remain the most popular blotting matrices for proteins and peptides. They are available from a number of suppliers including Schleicher and Schuell, Millipore and Bio-Rad. For most applications the 0.45 μm pore size membrane is recommended, although for proteins or peptides of <15 000 Da in size, the 0.2 μm pore size membrane has been reported to provide better sensitivity; presumably this is due to reduced passage of the protein/peptide through the matrix. The major drawback of nitrocellulose is its extreme fragility. To avoid breakage nitrocellulose should be cut with very sharp scissors and handled with great care at all times.

A number of other, less fragile, membranes, based on nylon or other synthetic polymers, are also available. These can be obtained from the same suppliers as nitrocellulose. Some of these membranes have been derivatized to permit covalent linkage between the membrane and the protein. However, such a linkage is seldom, if ever, required for standard protein blotting techniques.

It is becoming increasingly common to sequence proteins directly from the membrane following Western blotting from complex mixtures. If this is the aim, then the blotting membrane must be able to stand the harsh chemical environment encountered during the sequencing reactions. Polyvinylidene difluoride (PVDF) based membranes (e.g. Immobilon-P from Millipore) are the membranes of choice.

3.2 Western blotting

3.2.1 Gel electrophoresis

i. Apparatus

Many excellent gel electrophoresis kits are commercially available (for example, from Bio-Rad, Hoefer, and Pharmacia Biotech) in both standard and 'minigel' formats. In our experience the resolution of minigels is very close to that of larger gels, and yet they can be run in a fraction of the time (45 min as compared with 4–6 h). In addition, they are more economical with reagents and sample. The apparatus should be assembled and run in accordance with the manufacturer's instructions.

ii. Gel preparation

The most widely used buffer system for the electrophoresis of proteins is the discontinuous system developed by Laemmli (15). SDS is usually included in the sample and gel buffers. This detergent adheres to the protein, thereby denaturing it. The charge on the SDS swamps that of the protein, and therefore separation occurs on the basis of size alone. If SDS is omitted (native gel electrophoresis) separation will occur according to a combination of size, shape, and net charge. Dithiothreitol (DTT) is included in the sample buffer to reduce disulphide bonds. If this omitted, the presence of disulphide-linked complexes of the target protein will become apparent as a shift to a higher M_r relative to the M_r in the presence of reductant. *Protocol 5* gives the procedure for running reducing, denaturing gels. Omit the SDS and DTT from the running and/or gel buffers as required for non-denaturing and/or non-reducing gels.

Protocol 5. SDS gel electrophoresis

Reagents

- Stock acrylamide[a] solution: dissolve 150 g of acrylamide and 4 g of *bis*-acrylamide in 500 ml of water. Store solution in a dark bottle at 4 °C.

- Stock running gel solutions are prepared as follows and stored in a dark bottle at 4 °C:

Final acrylamide concentration

	7.5%	10.0%	12.5%	15.0%	17.5%
Stock acrylamide (ml)	7.5	10.0	12.5	15.0	17.5
1 M Tris–HCl, pH 8.8 (ml)	11.2	11.2	11.2	11.2	11.2
20% SDS (ml)	0.15	0.15	0.15	0.15	0.15
H₂O	11.15	8.65	6.15	3.65	1.15

- Stock stacking gel solution: mix 16.7 ml of stock acrylamide solution, 12.5 ml of 1 M Tris–HCl, pH 6.8, 0.5 ml of 20% (w/v) SDS, and 57 ml of distilled H₂O. Store in a dark bottle at 4 °C.
- Running buffer: dissolve 14.35 g of glycine, 3.03 g of Tris base, and 1.0 g of SDS in 1 litre (final volume) of distilled water.
- 5 × sample buffer: mix 0.77 g of DTT, 1.0 g

of SDS, 4.0 ml of 1 M Tris, pH 6.8, 5.0 ml of glycerol, and 300 µl of 0.2% (w/v) bromo-phenol blue (dissolved in ethanol). Make up to 20 ml with distilled H₂O.
- TEMED: *N,N,N′,N′*-tetramethylethylene-diamine
- 10% (w/v) ammonium persulphate, freshly prepared
- Water-saturated butan-1-ol

Method

1. Decant a suitable volume (typically 10 ml for two minigels) of stock running gel solution. For each 10 ml add 15 µl of TEMED and 100 µl of freshly prepared 10% ammonium persulphate to initiate polymerization.

2. Immediately pour the gel mix into the sealed, assembled plate apparatus allowing sufficient space (approximately 10% of the length of the gel) for the stacking gel.

3. Overlay the gel carefully with water-saturated butan-1-ol and allow to polymerize (approximately 30 min).

4. After the gel has polymerized, decant off the butan-1-ol and rinse the top of the gel with distilled water.

5. Overlay gel with a suitable volume (typically 5 ml for two minigels) of stock stacking gel solution. For each 5 ml add 15 µl of TEMED and 50 µl of freshly prepared ammonium persulphate.

Protocol 5. *Continued*

6. Immediately insert a clean comb and allow the gel to polymerize (approximately 15 min).

7. Assemble the polymerized gel into the electrophoresis apparatus according to manufacturer's instructions.

8. Fill the tank reservoirs with running buffer.

9. If the samples have not been prepared previously with 5 × sample buffer, add 0.25 volumes of 5 × sample buffer. Place in a boiling water bath for 2 min.[b]

10. Load the samples and connect the apparatus to a suitable power supply.

11. Apply current in accordance with the manufacturer's recommendations (200 V, constant voltage, for a Bio-Rad minigel) until the bromophenol blue in the samples has migrated to within 0.5 cm of the bottom of the gel.

---

[a] Note that acrylamide and *bis*-acrylamide are neurotoxins. Always wear gloves when handling either powder or solutions and avoid generating dust when weighing out.

[b] If clinical fluids are being analysed directly (see Section 2.4), centrifuge the boiled sample at 13 000 g for 5 min prior to use in order to pellet any debris.

Following electrophoresis, the gel can be used for electrophoretic transfer without further manipulation. Western blotting need not be restricted to gels run using the Laemmli buffer system; indeed, any acrylamide-based gel can be used. However, it is important to ensure that the conductivity of the gel is not excessive. Therefore when using gel systems with high ionic strength buffers, the gel should be equilibrated in transfer buffer (see *Protocol 6*) prior to electrophoretic transfer.

3.2.2 Electrophoretic transfer

Two types of electrophoretic transfer systems are available, termed 'wet' and 'semi-dry'. In the wet method, the gel and associated membrane are completely immersed in buffer. In the more recently developed semi-dry method, buffer-saturated filter papers serve as the ion reservoirs. One real advantage of semi-dry over wet blotting is the ease with which it can be used to blot multiple gels simultaneously. This is of great benefit if a high throughput of Western blots is required.

i. Wet blotting method

Commercial gel electrophoresis apparatus usually forms part of an integrated system which includes apparatus required for electrophoretic transfer. Given the large currents involved it is recommended that these systems are used because of their inbuilt safety features. Electrophoretic transfer using the wet method is described in *Protocol 6*.

Protocol 6. Wet Western blotting

Equipment and reagents

- Transfer buffer[a]
- Whatman 3MM filter paper
- Scotchbrite pads
- Transfer membrane (see Section 3.1)

Method

1. Cut four pieces of Whatman 3MM filter paper and one piece of transfer membrane to dimensions slightly larger than the gel and soak in transfer buffer.[a]

2. Place two pieces of the 3MM paper on top of a fibre pad (Scotchbrite; Bio-Rad).

3. Place the gel on top of the 3MM paper. Ensure that no air bubbles are trapped.

4. Place the transfer membrane on top of the gel. Ensure that all air bubbles are removed, as any bubbles trapped under the membrane will appear as white areas on the developed blot. Air bubbles can be removed by rolling a glass rod or pipette over the assembly.

5. Place the remaining two pieces of 3MM paper on top of the transfer membrane.

6. Complete the 'sandwich' by placing another fibre pad (Scotchbrite) on top of the filter paper (*Figure 2*).

7. Place the sandwich into the plastic support supplied by the manufacturer and place in the buffer tank in the correct orientation.[b]

8. Fill the tank with transfer buffer[a] and connect the apparatus to a power supply.

9. Apply the electric current in strict accordance with the manufacturer's guidelines.[c]

---

[a] Everybody has their favourite transfer buffer. We find the most convenient to be five volumes of 1 × Laemmli running buffer (see *Protocol 5*), three volumes of distilled water and two volumes of methanol. This buffer contains SDS which seems to improve the transfer of large and hydrophobic proteins. However, the SDS can be omitted if required. Some workers have found that using isopropanol in place of methanol improves transfer. For transfer to PVDF membranes (or for very basic proteins) 10 mM 3-[cyclohexylamino]-1-propanesulphonic acid pH 11.0 and 10% (v/v) methanol is recommended.

[b] If the blotting sandwich is assembled as described above (and as shown in *Figure 2*), the bottom of the sandwich represents the cathodic side, i.e. the side which should be inserted facing the negative electrode. The (negatively charged) proteins migrate towards the anode (*Figure 2*).

[c] Individual manufacturers of blotting equipment have their own guidelines on the length of time required for blotting, but this is likely to require some optimization. For minigels 30 min to 1 h is usually sufficient.

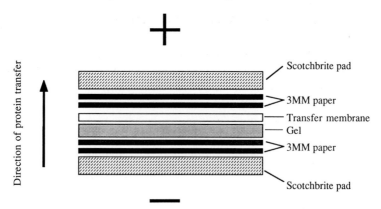

Figure 2. Assembly of a 'wet' transfer sandwich for electrophoresis. The procedure is described in detail in *Protocol 6*.

ii. Semi-dry blotting method

As with wet blotting, commercial equipment is available (for example, from Bio-Rad) and a variety of buffer systems can be used. We have found the buffer system described in *Protocol 7* to be the most satisfactory.

Protocol 7. Semi-dry Western blotting

Equipment and reagents

- Anode buffer 1: 0.3 M Tris, 10% (v/v) methanol, pH 10.4
- Anode buffer 2: 25 mM Tris, 10% (v/v) methanol, pH 10.4
- Cathode buffer: 25 mM Tris, 40 mM 6-aminohexanoic acid
- Whatman 3MM filter paper

Method

1. For each gel to be blotted cut one piece of transfer membrane and six pieces of Whatman 3MM filter paper to the same size as the gel.

2. Soak one piece of 3MM in anode buffer 1.

3. Allow excess buffer to drain from the filter paper and place on the lower electrode surface. In the case of semi-dry blotting this is the anode. Ensure that no air bubbles are trapped.

4. Soak, and then drain, two pieces of 3MM paper in anode buffer 2. Place on top of filter paper already in position.

5. Soak the transfer membrane in anode buffer 2 and place on top of the filter papers. Remove any trapped air bubbles with a glass rod or pipette as described in *Protocol 6*.

6. Place the gel on top of the transfer membrane. Ensure that no air bubbles are trapped.

---

7. Soak three pieces of 3MM paper in cathode buffer, drain, and place over the gel.

8. The assembly described above represents one transfer unit. If more than one gel is to be blotted then continue assembling transfer units on top of each other, but separate individual units with a sheet of dialysis membrane soaked in distilled water.

9. Place the top electrode (cathode) of the apparatus in position.

10. Apply an appropriate voltage in strict accordance with the manufacturer's guidelines.

3.2.3 Slot and dot blotting

Slot and dot blotting involve the direct application of the sample to be probed on to a membrane which has been masked by a template. Apparatus commonly has interchangeable templates for slot and dot blotting. Such equipment can be obtained from Schleicher and Schuell, Bio-Rad, and Millipore, amongst others. The apparatus is usually connected to a vacuum line which draws the sample through the membrane. Dot blot templates have 12 rows of eight holes arranged at the same spacings as 96-well microtitre plates whereas slot blot templates have up to 48 slots, aligned in rows. The slot blot arrangement of thin lines in rows is designed to facilitate densitometric analysis of the developed blot. Therefore slot blotting is particularly suited for quantitative measurements.

The apparatus should be assembled and used according to the manufacturer's instructions. The user should be aware that it can take a surprisingly long time for proteinaceous samples to be drawn through the small pores of the membrane.

3.3 Detection of protein following transfer

Following transfer it is useful to stain the membrane for protein. This achieves two things: firstly, the efficiency of the transfer can be evaluated, and secondly, a permanent record of the positions of the bands can be obtained, either on the filter itself, or as a photograph.

3.3.1 India ink staining

If the blot is to be probed with ^{125}I-labelled protein A or ^{125}I-labelled protein G, the filter can be permanently stained using India ink. However, this method is not suitable for colorimetric methods as the reaction product will be obscured by the staining. To stain with India ink, immerse the membrane in a solution containing 0.1% (v/v) Tween-20 and 0.1% (v/v) India ink. The protein will appear as a black stain on a grey background. Once the desired intensity has been achieved, wash the membrane with 0.1% (v/v) Tween-20.

The presence of the ink particles does not appear to have any significant effect on the immunoreactivity of the protein.

3.3.2 Ponceau S staining

For reversible staining of nitrocellulose stain the membrane for 1 min with a solution containing 0.5% (w/v) Ponceau S and 1% (v/v) acetic acid. Destain the nitrocellulose with water. The protein will be stained dark pink. If required the membrane can be photographed at this stage. The stain will be removed in the alkaline environment of the blocking buffer (see Section 3.4).

3.4 Blocking

Following the application of the sample and staining of the membrane it is necessary to block remaining protein-binding sites on the membrane. This is accomplished by soaking the membrane in a solution of protein. A number of proteins have been used for this purpose, including gelatin, casein, and bovine serum albumin (BSA). However, a blocking solution of 1% (w/v) dried non-fat (skimmed) milk and 0.5% (v/v) Triton X-100 in PBS appears to give the lowest background, is easy to prepare, and is economical to use. The membrane should be immersed and agitated in the blocking solution for at least 30 min.

3.5 Probing with primary antibody

Either polyclonal or monoclonal antibodies can be used as the primary antibody probe. The procedures used in blotting (see above) result in at least partial denaturation of the target species which may lead to the destruction of particular epitopes. It is therefore not uncommon to find monoclonal antibodies which do not react with blotted proteins. Human serum samples should be inactivated prior to use in order to ensure that any infectious virus is destroyed. The inactivation procedure will depend on the virus thought to be present. For HIV-positive samples, the serum can be inactivated either as described in *Protocol 1* or by heating at 56 °C for 2 h.

The optimal primary antibody dilution needs to be determined empirically. As a guideline, polyclonal serum can normally be used at 1:1000, hybridoma culture supernatants at 1:10 to 1:100, and murine ascites fluid at ≥1:1000. Dilute the antibody using blocking solution and place it along with the filter in a heat-sealable plastic bag. Attach the bag to a tube rotator or place on an orbital shaker for 30 min to 1 h. Remove the filter from the bag and wash in three changes of blocking solution for 3 min each.

3.6 Detecting bound antibody

Protocols for detecting the bound primary antibody are given below. The ^{125}I-labelled protein A/protein G and chemiluminescence systems result in the image being formed on a photographic film. The use of alkaline phosphatase or horseradish peroxidase conjugates results in visualization of the reaction directly on the membrane using a colorimetric substrate. Quantitative densitometry of films is much easier than densitometry of opaque membranes (which have to be densitometered in reflectance mode), and consequently the photographic systems should be considered if a quantitative value is required.

3.6.1 ^{125}I-labelled protein A or protein G

Protein A, which is isolated from the cell walls of *Staphylococcus aureus*, varies in the affinity with which it binds to immunoglobulins of different species. Whilst it binds to IgA and most IgG subclasses of many species, its binding to murine and avian immunoglobulins is poor. Protein G (isolated from Group G streptococci) binds more strongly to rat IgG than protein A, but does not bind to IgA. If protein G is used it is recommended that the recombinant version is used which is available from Pharmacia-LKB and has had the albumin binding domain removed. This will eliminate background reaction caused by the protein G binding to any albumin on the blot. *Protocol 8* describes the development of blots using ^{125}I-labelled protein A or ^{125}I-labelled protein G.

Protocol 8. Detection with ^{125}I-labelled protein A/protein G

Equipment and reagents

- ^{125}I-labelled protein A/protein G [a]
- Blocking buffer (see Section 3.4): 0.5% (w/v) dried non-fat milk and 0.5% (v/v) Triton X-100 in PBS (see *Protocol 2*)
- Whatman 3MM filter paper
- X-ray film

Method

1. Add 0.25 µCi of ^{125}I-labelled protein A (or ^{125}I-labelled protein G) per ml of blocking buffer.[b]

2. Place the solution into a heat-sealable bag along with the washed transfer membrane.

3. Place the assembly in a Pyrex dish and incubate on a rocking platform for 2–3 h.

4. Wash the transfer membrane with five or six changes of blocking buffer. Each wash should be for at least 3 min.

5. Drain the transfer membrane and place on a piece of 3MM filter paper cut slightly larger than the transfer membrane.

6. Wrap in plastic film.

7. Expose to X-ray film.

[a] To minimize exposure to ^{125}I, it is recommended that protein A/protein G is purchased already conjugated to [125]I (available from Amersham).
[b] Use approximately 5 ml/25 cm^2 transfer membrane.

3.6.2 Enzymatic detection of bound antibody

Bound antibody can be detected using secondary antibodies which have been raised against a specific immunoglobulin and conjugated to an enzyme. The enzymes most commonly used for conjugation are alkaline phosphatase and horseradish peroxidase. We have not found much to choose from between antibodies conjugated to either of these two enzymes, except that the horse-radish peroxidase reaction is quicker to develop. For most purposes, antibody–enzyme conjugates are available from commercial sources.

i. Alkaline phosphatase

The substrate used most frequently with alkaline phosphatase conjugated antibodies is bromochloroindolyl phosphate/nitro blue tetrazolium (BCIP/NBT). The insoluble precipitate produced at the site of antibody binding is an intense purple colour, giving a good level of contrast between the image and the membrane. *Protocol 9* describes the development of immunoblots with alkaline phosphatase conjugated antibody and BCIP/NBT.

Protocol 9. Detection with alkaline phosphatase

Reagents

- NBT solution: dissolve 0.5 g of NBT in 10 ml of 70% dimethylformamide.[a] Store at 4°C.
- BCIP solution: dissolve 0.5 g of BCIP (disodium salt) in 10 ml of 100% dimethylformamide. Store at 4°C.

- Alkaline phosphatase buffer: 100 mM NaCl, 5 mM $MgCl_2$, 100 mM Tris–HCl, pH 9.5
- PBS (see *Protocol 2*) containing 20 mM EDTA
- Tris-buffered saline (TBS): 150 mM NaCl, 50 mM Tris–HCl, pH 7.5

Method

1. Wash the blot in two changes of TBS for 3 min each.

2. Dilute the antibody–alkaline phosphatase conjugate in TBS containing 1% (w/v) non-fat dried milk. In general, conjugates are used at concentrations of approximately 0.5–5 μg/ml. For commercial preparations, this is usually a 1/200 to 1/2000 dilution.

3. Incubate the blot with the antibody solution inside a heat-sealed bag. Attach the bag to a tube rotator or orbital shaker for 1 h.

4. Wash the blot with three changes of TBS containing 1% (w/v) non-fat dried milk for 3 min each.

5. Prepare fresh substrate solution by adding 66 μl of NBT solution to 10 ml of alkaline phosphatase buffer. Mix well and add 33 μl of BCIP solution.

6. Add 5 ml of fresh substrate solution per 25 cm^2 of membrane. Develop the blot by agitating at room temperature until the bands are of the desired intensity. This usually takes approximately 30 min.

7. Stop the reaction by rinsing the blot in PBS containing 20 mM EDTA.

---

ii. Horseradish peroxidase

The three substrates most frequently reacted with horseradish peroxidase antibody conjugates are chloronaphthol, aminoethylcarbazole, and diamino-benzidine (DAB), which produce blue-black, red, and brown reaction products, respectively. The colour of the DAB reaction product can, however, be changed to blue-black by adding heavy metal salts. DAB is the most sensitive of the three substrates and is therefore the substrate of choice in our laboratory. *Protocol 10* describes the development of immunoblots using horseradish peroxidase conjugates and DAB.

Horseradish peroxidase conjugated antibodies can also be used for chemiluminescence detection. Horseradish peroxidase is used to catalyse the oxidation of diacylhydrazides, such as luminol, to produce an excited state which may then decay to the ground state via a light-emitting pathway. Consequently, the signal is detected on photographic film. Horseradish peroxidase bound to a blot in any configuration (see below) can be used for this type of reaction. The required substrates are available in kit form (Amersham) and come complete with a comprehensive protocol.

Protocol 10. Detection with horseradish peroxidase

Reagents

- Blocking buffer: see *Protocol 8*
- 50 mM sodium phosphate buffer, pH 7.4
- 2.5% (w/v) DAB dissolved in PBS (see *Protocol 2*).[a] The DAB solution can be stored in aliquots at −20 °C.
- A solution containing 1% (w/v) cobalt chloride and 1% (w/v) ammonium nickel sulphate
- 30% solution of hydrogen peroxide

Method

1. Dilute the antibody–horseradish peroxidase conjugate in blocking buffer (see step 2, *Protocol 9*).

2. Incubate the blot for 1 h with the antibody solution inside a heat-sealed bag as described in *Protocol 9*, step 3.

3. Wash the blot in a suitable container with three changes of blocking buffer for 3 min each.

4. Prepare fresh substrate solution by mixing the following:
   - 25 ml of 50 mM sodium phosphate buffer. pH 7.4
   - 400 μl of 2.5% DAB solution
   - 0.5 ml of the cobalt chloride/ammonium nickel sulphate solution
   - 50 μl of 30% hydrogen peroxide

   The heavy metal solution should be added dropwise. A small precipitate will form, but this does not adversely affect the reaction.

Protocol 10. *Continued*

5. Add 5 ml of fresh substrate solution per 25 cm^2 of membrane. Develop the blot by agitating at room temperature until the bands are of the desired intensity. This usually takes approximately 3–5 min.

6 Stop the reaction by rinsing the blot in distilled H$_2$O.

---

^{a} Some chromogenic substrates (for example, DAB) may be carcinogenic and should be handled accordingly.

3.7 Increasing sensitivity

For the detection systems described above, the limit of detection is approximately 20 fmol. For a 50 000 Da protein, this represents about 1 ng. To detect proteins present at lower abundance, concentration of the target species, perhaps by partial purification of the protein, may be required. The intensity of the signal obtained in blotting analyses can be increased to some extent by improving the detection system used. Three main approaches have been used to increase sensitivity, all of which rely on increasing the size of the immune complex (*Figure 3*) (16–18). It should be noted, however, that increasing the sensitivity can also result in increasing background reactions and a balance must therefore be found between the two.

3.7.1 Triple layers

The number of labelled molecules bound to the antigen can be increased by using a non-labelled secondary antibody followed by a third, labelled antibody raised against the species immunoglobulin used as the secondary

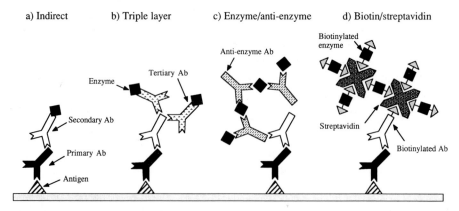

Figure 3. Procedures used to increase the sensitivity of Western and dot/slot blots, (a) Indirect standard procedure (*Protocol 9*); (b) triple layer of antibodies (see Section 3.7.1); (c) enzyme–anti-enzyme complex (see Section 3.7.2); (d) biotin–streptavidin complexes (see Section 3.7.3).

antibody (*Figure 3*b). An amplification of the signal results from the fact that more than one anti-immunoglobulin antibody can bind to the primary and secondary antibodies.

3.7.2 Enzyme/anti-enzyme complexes

In this method, amplification is achieved by using an enzyme/anti-enzyme complex which is linked to the primary antibody using an anti-immunoglobulin bridging antibody (*Figure 3*c) (16). The most frequently used complex is peroxidase/anti-peroxidase which is available commercially (Sigma). It is important to remember that the species used to raise the primary antibody and the anti-peroxidase antibody must be the same.

3.7.3 Biotin–streptavidin complexes

Increased sensitivity using biotin–streptavidin complexes is based on the fact that each streptavidin (or avidin) molecule can bind four biotin molecules. The biotin–streptavidin complex is formed by mixing streptavidin with an enzyme which has previously been biotinylated. The complex is prepared such that there are still biotin-binding sites available on the streptavidin molecules. This large biotin-binding, enzymatically active complex is used to detect antigen either via a directly biotinylated primary antibody or via a biotinylated anti-immunoglobulin second antibody (*Figure 3*d) (17, 18).

4. Applications

Blotting procedures can be used to determine a range of important character-istics of both antibodies and antigens. The principal advantage of these methods is that antigens are available on a membrane for probing with antibodies (or other ligands) rather than being inaccessible within a gel. The use of blotting techniques to examine the reactivity pattern of a patient's antibodies against a particular virus may eventually lead to new methods of disease monitoring and diagnosis, in addition to providing a better under-standing of the interaction between the infectious agent itself and the immune response it elicits. Advances in dot and slot blotting techniques, combined with the availability of monoclonal antibodies or recombinant proteins and peptides, should result in further development of new and rapid diagnostic tests for use in both field testing centres and clinical laboratories.

The main applications of blotting procedures, with particular reference to use in the field of medical virology are summarized below.

(a) A major use of blotting techniques in virology is as a confirmatory test to detect infection with a particular virus. Probably the best known con-firmatory assays are the Western blots used for detecting antibodies to HIV, HTLV-I, and HCV proteins in serum samples (1–4). The scope of this type of assay can also be extended to differential diagnosis of clinical samples by using antigens derived from different viral isolates. For example, type 1 and type 2 HIV infections can be distinguished by using Western blot strips loaded with proteins derived from HIV-1- or HIV-2-infected cell cultures (19).

(b) Dot and slot blotting procedures can also be used for detecting antibodies in clinical samples. These techniques have been used recently to develop assays using recombinant proteins (7) and peptides (Peptilav-1–2, Diagnostics Pasteur). For example, in HIV infections the reactivity of antibodies in polyclonal sera with specific regions of certain viral proteins is often of interest. Using a dot or slot blot format, it is possible to design an assay strip containing multiple antigens at defined locations. This can then be used for detecting specific antibodies within a polyclonal serum sample in a single test. An additional advantage is that HIV-1 and HIV-2 antigens can be loaded on to the same test strip, thereby allowing differential diagnosis in one assay (see *Figure 4*). Specific examples where Western blotting or dot/slot blotting have been used to characterize human viral pathogens are shown in *Table 1*.

(c) The amount of antibody binding to a specific antigen can be quantified in either Western blots or dot/slot blots using either radiolabelled or chemiluminescent detection systems (29).

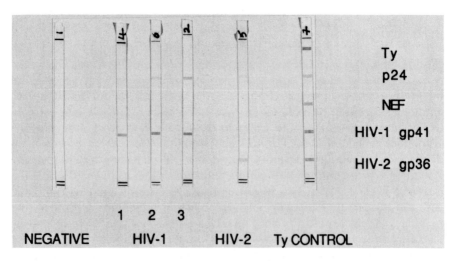

Figure 4. Reactivity of HIV-1 and HIV-2 sera with recombinant Ty virus-like particle (Ty-VLP) antigens. Recombinant hybrid proteins were produced by fusing HIV gene fragments to the *TYA* gene of the yeast retrotransposon Ty. The fragments contained regions of the *gag* p24, *nef*, and gp41 genes of HIV-1 and the gp36 gene of HIV-2. The resulting fusion proteins assembled into virus-like particles and were purified and loaded on to nitrocellulose strips in a slot blot format (reference 7). The strips were probed with antisera against HIV-1, HIV-2, or recombinant Ty-VLPs (Ty control). The reactivities of HIV-1- and HIV-2-positive sera can be clearly distinguished.

Table 1. Use of protein blotting to characterize human viral pathogens

Virus	Family	Reference
BK virus	Papovaviridae	20
Cytomegalovirus	Herpesviridae	21
Epstein–Barr virus	Herpesviridae	22
Hepatitis B virus	Hepadnaviridae	23
Hepatitis C virus	Not classified	4
Herpes simplex virus	Herpesviridae	24
HIV	Retroviridae	1, 2, 5–7
HTLV-I	Retroviridae	3
Japanese encephalitis virus	Flaviviridae	25
Respiratory syncytial virus	Paramyxoviridae	26
Rotavirus	Reoviridae	27
Varicella-zoster virus	Herpesviridae	28

(d) As with other immunoassays such as ELISAs, the isotype of the binding antibody can be determined by using different isotype-specific secondary antibodies in the detection system. The use of a dot/slot blot format for such studies may be advantageous when screening multiple samples for immunoglobulin class and subclass (30).

(e) Both Western blotting and dot/slot blotting techniques can be used to determine the binding specificities of monoclonal antibodies. Dot/slot blotting procedures may be particularly useful when a large number of antibodies are to be screened or if the antibodies do not detect denatured antigens (31).

(f) Blotting procedures can be used to determine the level of expression of recombinant viral proteins (32, 33). In addition, they can be used to evaluate the effect of specific mutations on the binding ability of monoclonal antibodies. Such mutational analyses could facilitate the identification of, for example, important antigenic determinants, receptor binding sites or active sites of viral enzymes (34).

(g) Western blot assays can be used to evaluate the specificity of antiviral compounds. For example, if a specific viral protease cleaves other viral polyproteins, the inhibition of cleavage by a particular antiviral compound could be monitored by separating the reaction products on an SDS–polyacrylamide gel followed by detection of the cleaved and/or non-cleaved proteins using specific antibodies (35).

(h) Techniques are available for sequencing proteins immobilized on blotting membranes (36). It is therefore possible to determine the sequence of viral proteins from a mixture following Western blotting, thereby avoiding the need to develop purification procedures for each individual protein of interest.

(i) Antibodies in polyclonal sera reactive with a particular protein band can be purified by eluting the antibody after binding (37). The electrophoresis and transfer are carried out as usual, but with the same sample loaded across the gel. After incubation with the primary antibody, the end tracks of the blot are developed and bound antibody is detected as normal. This allows the protein of interest on the rest of the filter to be located. The area of the blot that contains the antigen and primary antibody is excised from the filter and the antibody eluted with 100 mM glycine (pH 2.5). The solution is then removed from the filter strip and neutralized with a 0.1 volume of 1 M Tris-HCl (pH 8.0).

References

1. Martin, P. W., Burger, D. R., Caoutte, S., Goldstein, A. S., and Peetoom, F. (1986). *N. Engl. J. Med.*, **317**, 1577.
2. Thorpe, R., Brasher, M. D., Bird, C. R., Garrett, A. J., Jacobs, J. P., Minor, P. D., and Schild, G. C. (1987). *J. Virol. Methods*, **16**, 87.
3. Centers for Disease Control (1988). *Morbid. Mortal. Weekly Rep.*, **37**, 736.
4. Janot, C. and Courouce, A. M. (1990). *Rev. Fr. Transfus. Hemobiol.*, **33**, 439.
5. Blumberg, R. S., Hartshorn, K. L., Ardman, B., Kaplan, J. C., Paradis, T., Vogt, M., *et al.* (1987). *J. Clin. Microbiol.*, **25**, 1989.
6. Little, D. and Ferris, J. A. (1990). *J. Forensic Sci.*, **35**, 1029.
7. Gilmour, J. E. M., Read, S. J., Eglin, R., Ryan, C., Burns, N. R., Graff, N., *et al.* (1990). *AIDS*, **4**, 967.
8. Corey, L. (1986). *Diagn. Microbiol. Infect. Dis.*, **4**, 1115.
9. Fields, B. N. and Knipe, D. M. (ed.) (1990). *Virology*. Raven Press, New York.
10. Goeddel, D. V. (ed.) (1990). *Methods in enzymology*, Vol. 185. Academic Press, London.
11. Deutscher, M. P. (ed.) (1990). *Methods in enzymology*, Vol. 182. Academic Press, London.
12. Lukow, V. A. and Summers, M. D. (1988). *Bio/Technology*, **6**, 47.
13. Towbin, H., Staehelin, T., and Gordon, J. (1979). *Proc. Natl. Acad. Sci. USA*, **76**, 4350.
14. Burnette, W. N. (1981). *Anal. Biochem.*, **112**, 195.
15. Laemmli, U. K. (1970). *Nature*, **227**, 680.
16. Frazer, H. E. and Wisdom, G. B. (1985). *J. Immunol. Methods*, **8**, 221.
17. Bayer, E. A., Skutelsky, E., and Wilchek, M. (1979). *Methods in enzymology*, Vol. **62**, pp. 308–15. Academic Press, London.
18. Wilchek, M. and Bayer, E. A. (1984). *Immunology Today*, **5**, 39.
19. Clavel, F. (1987). *AIDS*, **1**, 135.
20. Christie, K. E., Flaegstad, T., and Traavik, T. (1988). *J. Med. Virol.*, **24**, 183.
21. Landini, M. P., Re, M. C., Mirolo, G., Baldassarri, B., and La Placa, M. (1985). *J. Med. Virol.*, **17**, 303.
22. Lin, J. C., Choi, E. I., and Pagano, J. S. (1985). *J. Virol.*, **53**, 793.
23. Pillot, J. and Petit, M. A. (1984). *Mol. Immunol.*, **21**, 53.
24. Lehtinen, M. (1985). *Ann. Clin. Res.*, **17**, 66.

25. Srivastava, A. K., Aira, Y., Mori, C., Kobayashi, Y., and Igarashi, A. (1987). *Arch. Virol.*, **96**, 97.
26. Routledge, E. G., Willcocks, M. M., Morgan, L., Samson, A. C., Scott, R., and Toms, G. L. (1987). *J. Gen. Virol.*, **68**, 1209.
27. Battaglia, M., Passarani, N., Di Matteo, A., and Gerna, G. (1987). *J. Infect. Dis.*, **155**, 140.
28. Harper, D. R., Kangro, H. O., and Heath, R. B. (1990). *J. Med. Virol.*, **30**, 61.
29. Schneppeheim, R. and Rautenberg, P. (1987). *Eur. J. Clin. Microbiol.*, **6**, 49.
30. Hawkes, R. (1986). *Methods in enzymology*, Vol. 121, pp. 484–91. Academic Press, London.
31. Bennett, F. C. and Yeoman, L. C. (1983). *J. Immunol. Methods*, **61**, 201.
32. Cabradilla, C. D., Groopman, J. E., Lanigan, J., Renz, M., Lasky, L. A., and Capon, D. J. (1986). *Biotechnology*, **4**, 128.
33. Mills, H. R., Berry, N., Burns, N. R., and Jones, I. M. (1992). *AIDS*, **6**, 437.
34. Samson, A. C. (1986). *J. Gen. Virol.*, **67**, 1199.
35. Baboonian, C., Dalgleish, A., Bountiff, L., Gross, J., Oroszlan, S., Rickett, G., *et al.* (1991). *Biochem. Biophys. Res. Commun.*, **179**, 17.
36. Vandekerckhove, J., Bauw, G., Puype, M., Van Damme, J., and Van Montagu, M. (1985). *Eur. J. Biochem.*, **152**, 9.
37. Olmsted, J. B. (1981). *J. Biol. Chem.*, **256**, 11955.

5

Polymerase chain reaction

P. SIMMONDS

1. Principles of the polymerase chain reaction

The polymerase chain reaction (PCR) provides the means to amplify specific sequences of DNA an essentially unlimited number of times. The method was first used to amplify human DNA sequences (1–4) and since then has been used extensively as an alternative or an adjunct to cloning in bacterial vectors for analysis of eukaryotic and prokaryotic genomes. It was quickly realized that the PCR also provided the means to amplify viral nucleic acid sequences present in virus cultures or directly from clinical specimens (5, 6), and thus could provide a highly sensitive and specific general detection system for any virus for which there were sufficient nucleotide sequence data to produce virus-specific primers. In this chapter, the principles of the PCR are briefly explained, followed by a series of recommendations concerning how PCR may be set up in a diagnostic virology laboratory, and how problems of contamination may be avoided. This is followed by detailed protocols for extraction of DNA and RNA from clinical specimens, reverse transcription of RNA, the PCR method itself, and two methods for sensitive and specific detection of the amplified DNA. The emphasis in this chapter is on optimizing the PCR for sensitivity and reproducibility; in the space provided, it has not proved possible to provide practical information on the analysis of amplified viral DNA, such as restriction endonuclease cleavage and nucleotide sequencing. However, a series of references to publications that describe the differentiation and typing of different viral strains and types is given.

1.1 Mechanism of the amplification reaction (*Figure 1*)

The PCR method is ultimately dependent on primer-initiated DNA synthesis, since DNA replicating enzymes normally require a short section of double-stranded DNA on a single-stranded template to 'prime' DNA copying. Following increased automation in nucleic acid chemistry, it is now possible to synthesize short pieces of single-stranded DNA of defined sequence (oligonucleotides). In appropriate conditions, sequence-specific binding of an

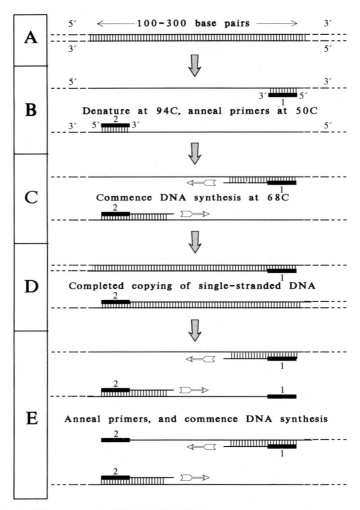

Figure 1. Amplification of viral DNA by PCR. (A) Sample heated to 94 °C to denature DNA and separate strands. (B) Sample cooled to 50 °C, to allow hybridization of primers to target sequences approximately 100–300 base pairs apart on opposite strands. (C) Sample warmed to 68 °C to commence DNA synthesis on each strand from the two primers in opposite directions. (D) Completion of synthesis. (E) Second cycle: denaturation followed by annealing of primers to two original strands of viral DNA and to the two copied strands of DNA. DNA synthesis initiated to generate four copies of viral sequence. In the third cycle (not shown), each of the eight sequences will again be copied. PCR was continued for 25 heating cycles (not shown).

oligonucleotide to 'target' DNA by hydrogen bonding between matched base-pairs (hybridization) will take place. This short stretch of double-stranded DNA will now serve as the initiation point for DNA replication by polymerase enzymes (*Figure 1b*). In the PCR, two oligonucleotide 'primers' are used, one complementary in sequence to one strand of DNA, and the other complementary to a DNA sequence on the other strand several hundred base-pairs away. DNA synthesis is initiated by the two oligonucleotides in opposite directions (*Figure 1c*), and will eventually replicate the recognition site of the opposite primer (*Figure 1d*).

By alternately heating and cooling the reaction mixture, it is possible to obtain exponential amplification of DNA sequences between the primer binding sites (*Figure 1e*). Heating the sample to over 90°C denatures the DNA and separates the strands. On cooling to around 50°C, the primers hybridize to their complementary sequences and thereby initiate copying of the single-stranded template. The 'primer extension' reaction is normally carried out at around 70°C, which is the optimum temperature for heat-stable DNA polymerases now used in the PCR. Once this first cycle is completed, the sample is heated again to enable a further round of DNA amplification to take place. It can be seen from the relative position and orientation of the primers used for amplification not only that the original target sequence can be repeatedly copied by each heating cycle, but also that the product itself also serves as a template for further amplification. Thus, starting from a hypothetical single target sequence, the first heat cycle produces a copy of each strand. The second cycle again produces two copies from the original target DNA, and two further copies from the product of the first reaction. The third cycle produces copies from the original, copies from the two first PCR products, and copies from the four second PCR products, and so on. Thus, under ideal conditions, each heat cycle doubles the number of copies of the DNA sequence that lies between the two primers; thus after n cycles, in theory 2^n copies of product DNA are produced from each copy of target sequence (see below).

The first PCR protocols used DNA polymerase I (Klenow fragment) from *Escherichia coli* for copying of DNA (1–5). However, the high temperatures necessary for denaturation of DNA rapidly inactivated the enzyme, which therefore had to be replaced in every cycle. More recently, the DNA polymerase from the thermophilic bacterium, *Thermus aquaticus*, isolated from a hot spring in Yellowstone National Park and capable of growth at 70–75°C (7), has been used in the PCR (6, 8). This enzyme (*Taq* polymerase) is extremely resistant to thermal inactivation, and therefore does not need to be replaced during heat cycling. This has considerably simplified the PCR method and greatly improved its sensitivity and specificity. Since then other thermostable DNA polymerases have been used in the PCR, e.g. *Tth* polymerase from *Thermus thermophilus* (9), 'Vent' polymerase from *Thermococcus litoralis*, and *Pfu* polymerase from *Pyrococcus furiosus* (10), an extreme thermophile isolated from hot springs near Volcano in Italy. This bacterium thrives at even higher temperatures than *T. aquaticus* (around 100°C), and its DNA polymerase shows less thermal denaturation during the PCR than the *Taq* polymerase (11).

P. Simmonds

1.2 Limitations of and problems with the PCR

Having explained the basic principles by which the amplification reaction takes place, I will in the rest of the chapter describe the practical aspects of using this assay for detection of viral sequences in clinical material, the limitations of the method, and the situations where it does or could find clinical application.

According to the scheme outlined above, one might expect that, given sufficient heat cycles, it would be possible to achieve unlimited amplification from as little as a single molecule of target DNA. The amount of product can be calculated according to the following formula:

$$\text{product} = \frac{2^n \times l \times m}{A}$$

where n is the number of heat cycles, l the length of amplified fragment (in base pairs), m the average mass of a base pair (constant), and A Avogadro's number, 6×10^{23}.

For example, if a single molecule of target sequence was amplified with primers spaced 500 bp apart over 10 cycles, the amount of DNA produced would be:

$$\frac{2^{10} \times 500 \times 660 \text{ g/mol}}{6 \times 10^{23}/\text{mol}} = 520 \text{ ag } (1 \text{ ag} = 10^{-18} \text{ g})$$

Substituting larger numbers of cycles into the equation shows that one might expect 580 fg after 20 cycles, 590 pg after 30 cycles, and finally 610 ng (0.61 µg) after 40 cycles. This latter amount would be readily detectable by agarose gel electrophoresis of the PCR product, followed by ethidium bromide staining.

However, there are limits to the degree of amplification possible using the unmodified method described above, and severe constraints on the specificity of the amplification reaction. Both of these problems prevent straightforward detection of amplified DNA from the often extremely low amounts of viral genomes present in clinical material. To maximize the sensitivity of the PCR, a series of optimization procedures for the amplification reaction has been described, and more sensitive and specific methods for detection of the amplified product have been developed.

To understand what limits the degree and specificity of PCR, it is necessary to consider the mechanics of the reaction in more detail. A necessity for the reaction is that during the 'cold' part of the cycle, the virus-specific primer hybridizes only to the target sequence for which it was designed. However, in complex DNA, such as human genomic DNA present in the clinical sample, there may, by chance, exist sequences that partially match the viral sequence, and which may under certain conditions hybridize with the PCR primer. Although such mis-pairing is not favoured, once it occurs, the mismatched DNA will be rapidly stabilized by the extension reaction. The likelihood of non-target DNA primed DNA replication depends principally on its complexity, in that the larger the number of different combinations of bases, the more likely will be the possibility of a partial match with the primers used for PCR (the haploid human genome contains approximately 3×10^9 bases, and will interfere significantly with amplification). The degree of non-specific amplification also depends on the amount on non-target DNA present in the sample being amplified, on the precise reaction conditions used in the PCR (particularly the stringency of the annealing step (see Section 4.4.1)), and on the number of cycles employed during the PCR.

Adventitious priming of DNA replication in itself does not necessarily cause any problems, and inevitably occurs to a greater or lesser extent during any amplification procedure. The problems start when one of the mis-primed copies of non-target DNA is in turn mis-primed and thus replicated in the opposite direction by a second primer. The product will comprise non-target DNA in the centre flanked by perfect matches to one or other primer at each end. This 'hybrid' DNA may now be amplified as effectively as true target DNA. Primer dimers are very short hybrid sequences, consisting entirely of two primer sequences fused together and capable of rapid replication under PCR conditions. The appearance of non-target hybrid DNA is probably the main limiting factor governing the yield of product, and one which limits the length of DNA that can be successfully amplified by PCR.

1.3 Selection of primers

The PCR is capable of amplifying the whole range of viral genomes. Examination of *Figure 1* shows that single-stranded DNA target sequences can also be amplified, even though only one of the two primers is actually used in the first PCR cycle. By incorporating a reverse transcription step prior to amplification by PCR (*Protocol 3*), it is possible to amplify cDNA copies of single- and double-stranded RNA genomes. The following general points should be considered when specifying primers:

1.3.1 Primer sequences

(a) Primers should normally have a minimum length of 17 or 18 bases, since shorter sequences than this are more likely to match non-viral sequences. DNA the size of the human genome can contain every combination of up to 16 bases. Although the human genome is largely comprised of repetitive DNA sequences, with far fewer combinations of bases than the maximum, the possibility of priming of DNA replication with mis-paired primers (see above) requires the above margin of safety. Primers longer than 28 bases should also be avoided as they can also cause non-specific annealing at the temperatures normally used for PCR (see Section 4.4.1). For example, specific annealing with a 30 base primer can only be obtained at temperatures around 80 °C, which is well above the optimum temperature for DNA replication by *Taq* polymerase.

(b) The strength of binding of primers to target DNA depends on G+C content, as G forms three hydrogen bonds with C, compared with only two between A and T (Section 4.4.1). For this reason, it is recommended that the primer sequence should contain at least 45% G+C. Furthermore, G+C-rich primers are less likely to hybridize to human genomic DNA which has a high A+T content (60%), and thus cause less non-specific amplification in the PCR.

(c) Runs of more than four or five of the same base in a primer should be avoided. In particular, primers containing many consecutive Gs are difficult to synthesize and purify.

(d) A primer sequence that could form secondary structures (i.e. complementarity of the ends leading to dimers or 'hairpins') should be avoided, as this will destabilize binding to its target sequence, and may lead to excessive primer dimer formation during the PCR.

(e) It is rarely necessary to size-purify the primer by high performance liquid chromatography (HPLC) before using in the PCR unless the primer is exceptionally long, or is to be used for sequencing. HPLC purification is also required when carrying out analysis of the PCR product by high resolution gel electrophoresis for size variation (e.g. as in reference 12) or restriction site polymorphisms, as the presence of shorter, imperfectly synthesized oligonucleotides will lead to heterogeneity in the size of the PCR product.

1.3.2 Avoidance of mismatches between primer and target sequences

Many viruses show considerable sequence heterogeneity, and to amplify all variants effectively, it is essential that the primer sites chosen are well conserved amongst all variants likely to be present in the clinical specimen to be amplified. For many viruses, e.g. hepatitis B virus (HBV) and human immunodeficiency virus type 1 (HIV-1), there is a wealth of comparative sequence data on which to base one's decision; for less well characterized viruses, particularly those with RNA genomes (which are almost always more variable than DNA viruses), there may be considerable problems. The following steps will help to minimize the risk of mismatches preventing detection of the intended range of viruses in the (usual!) situation of having only limited sequence data on which to base the primers.

(a) Mismatches at the downstream end of the primer, particularly the final base, affect the efficiency of amplification more than mismatches at the upstream end.

(b) Certain regions of the viral genome that encode capsid proteins, or those that have defined enzymatic functions (such as the *gag* and *pol* regions of retroviruses) are generally conserved to a higher degree than proteins encoding external membrane proteins (such as the *env* gene, reference

13). To improve the rate of detection of variants of such variable viruses, it is advisable to specify primers in such conserved regions to avoid mismatches.

(c) Regions encoding conserved viral proteins often contain a preponderance of silent substitutions (i.e. those that do not affect the amino acid sequence). It is a good general principle to ensure that the final base of the primer is not at such a 'silent' site, and if at all possible, the final 3–6 bases could correspond to codons with no alternatives (such as methionine (ATG) or tryptophan (TGG)).

(d) If it is suspected that mismatches may occur or cannot be avoided, primers can be made longer, so that the effect of mismatches on the overall stability of the primer–target DNA duplex is lessened. However, such primers may cause more non-specific amplification of non-target DNA (Section 1.3.1).

(e) To match variable residues in the viral sequence, it is possible to use inosine residues (which base-pair with A, C, or T), or to specify sites that contain two, three, or four different bases in the corresponding primer sequence. However, the use of such sites should be limited to avoid amplification of non-target DNA.

(f) As a general (empirical) principle, if primers match two distantly related viruses (such as HIV-1 and HIV-2), one may reasonably expect that they will also match variants of each virus type (i.e. all HIV-1 variants, and all HIV-2 variants).

1.3.3 Type-specific primers

There may well be occasions when it is necessary to distinguish between two related viruses. Although this may be achieved by the use of primers that amplify all variants followed by restriction enzyme or sequence analysis of the amplified DNA (Section 5.1), type-specific primers that are chosen deliberately to match one variant, and mismatch others may also be used. When specifying such primers, the following considerations should be borne in mind:

(a) Mismatches are only effective at the downstream end of the primer.

(b) To reduce amplification significantly, at least two and ideally more than four bases at the downstream end of the primer should be mismatched with the variant sequence.

(c) Differentiation of viruses by 'type-specific' primers is concentration dependent. Thus amplification of a mismatched variant may occur if present in large enough amounts.

(d) Primer sites that are suitable for differentiating types are often highly variable within the type itself. As the method is critically dependent on the degree of mismatch, variation within a type could significantly influence the results.

For further information, the reader is referred to publications in which methods for typing human papillomavirus (HPV) (14, 15), herpes simplex virus (16), HBV (17), and rotavirus (18) are described.

2. Sample preparation

2.1 Design of laboratory space and avoidance of contamination

It is a considerable commitment for a clinical virology laboratory to offer PCR as a diagnostic service. The techniques are generally unfamiliar to virology staff and require investment in new equipment. The problem that bedevils PCR detection is contamination of clinical specimens, buffers, and equipment with exogenous DNA (19), giving rise to false positive reactions (the three main sources of contaminating DNA in a laboratory are described in Section 4.2.3). The risk of contamination greatly increases with throughput of specimens, and it is essential that precautions are taken to avoid problems developing. Avoidance of contamination is the most important factor to consider in decisions as to where equipment is placed, and how samples are stored. Ideally, two or three separate rooms should be used to carry out PCR-related work, in addition to space required in the general laboratory for analysis of amplified DNA. These are:

- 'clean room' for storage and preparation of reagents for PCR
- sample preparation room for extraction of nucleic acids from clinical specimens
- PCR room for setting up reverse transcription and amplification reactions

The following sections list essential equipment and outline the stages to be carried out in each room.

2.1.1 'Clean' room

This room should be reserved for the preparation and storage of solutions, chemicals, reagents, and enzymes necessary for the PCR work. Pipette tips should also be placed in racks in this room. Essential items of equipment that should not be shared with other laboratories are as follows:

- $-20\,°C$ storage of enzymes, buffers etc.
- a full set of pipettes bought specifically for the purpose, and not used anywhere else (see below)
- a 0.5–1.5 ml tube microcentrifuge
- a vortex mixer

The following precautions should ensure that contamination of PCRs is avoided:

(a) Work should be carried out on a designated bench that should not be used for any other purpose.

(b) The work surface should be renewed at regular intervals to avoid contamination. (Sheets of disposable paper discarded after use, are a suitable bench-cover for this purpose.)

(c) Laboratory coats should not be worn outside of the designated room. Gloves should be discarded on leaving the room, and new ones put on on return.

(d) Departmental distilled water supplies often become contaminated with viral DNA from contact with the tap when filling beakers and bottles. As the volumes required for PCR are extremely small, it is usually worthwhile buying in pure water from a chemical supplier.

(e) Stocks of primers, nucleotide triphosphates, and PCR and reverse transcription (RT) buffers should be aliquoted and stored at $-20\,°C$. All aliquots and tubes of enzymes should be used one at a time. After thawing, tubes should be pulse-spun in a microcentrifuge to remove liquid adhering to the lid of the tube. Most suppliers of *Taq* polymerase and reverse transcriptase supply their own reaction buffers, and use of these reduces the risk of contamination associated with weighing out chemicals elsewhere in the department.

(f) Autoclaves used to treat waste material can become contaminated with viral DNA, and should not be used for sterilization of tips or tubes used for clinical specimens. Either a separate autoclave, or sterile pre-packed tips and tubes should be used.

2.1.2 Sample preparation

Extraction of viral nucleic acids from clinical specimens requires an environment that offers an appropriate level of safety for the operator, but also prevents contamination of the sample from exogenous DNA. For the majority of samples, handling in a Category 2 containment laboratory in a Class II microbiological safety hood that has been approved for use with pathogenic viruses is ideal (Class I hoods draw in unfiltered air and can lead to contamination of samples). For many viruses, it is permissible to use still-air cabinets. Handling samples on the open bench increases the risk of air-borne contamination by exogenous DNA.

i. Equipment

The following items are necessary for routine extraction of DNA and RNA from clinical specimens, and their use should be reserved for this purpose.

- low speed refrigerated centrifuge for pelleting of cells in transport medium, separation of peripheral blood mononuclear cells on Ficoll, clarification of plasma and serum
- medium speed refrigerated microcentrifuge for spinning 0.5 or 1.5 ml tubes at $10000\,g$ during DNA and RNA extraction

- optionally, an ultracentrifuge rotor for pelleting of virus from plasma or other biological fluids may be found necessary for some routine PCR work (for safety, rotors that take sealed swing-out tubes are preferable, although the number of samples that can be processed is considerably smaller than possible with some designs of fixed-angle rotors)
- a complete set of pipettes (2–20 µl, 10–100 µl, 20–200 µl, and 100–1000 µl), and racked boxes of tips of appropriate sizes (see below for precautions when using pipettes)
- an incubator, such as a thermostatically controlled hot-block, is necessary for many DNA and RNA extraction protocols

ii. Precautions

(a) Ideally, the room, and more particularly the containment hood, should not be used for purposes other than nucleic acid preparation. After use, it should be emptied of all items, and working surfaces swabbed to reduce the risk of subsequent contamination (see (h)). An ultraviolet light, if fitted, may also have some effect in reducing contamination (20).

(b) Apart from the above items of dedicated equipment, it is necessary to ensure that the laboratory is fully provided with consumables. These should be kept in cupboards in closed containers when not in use.

(c) Gloves should be used at all times. If the operator leaves the room, the gloves should be discarded on exit, and replaced on return (since viral DNA on door handles, freezer lids, etc. can lead to contamination of samples).

(d) Laboratory coats should be reserved for use in the sample preparation room and should be kept in the room when not in use.

(e) Care should be taken with the disposal of waste samples and plastic. Used plastic pipette tips and tubes should be immersed in a suitable de-contaminating solution (e.g. 2% glutaraldehyde or proprietary disinfectant, such as Tegodur) for the recommended time before disposal. Used disinfectant should be carefully discarded and splashing avoided.

(f) Positive displacement pipettes have often been recommended for PCR work (19), but have the disadvantage of requiring (relatively) expensive sealed tips. However, this author has not encountered problems with the conventional type, provided samples are pipetted slowly and are not mixed by a violent repetitive pipetting action, and that only the lower range of sample volumes is used with each pipette (to avoid fluid coming too close to the pipette barrel). Splashing of the barrel is more likely with the larger pipettes, and particular care should be exercised with the 1000 µl size. Pipettes larger than this should not be used. Tips should be racked outside of the sample preparation room on a bench reserved for preparation and aliquoting of PCR reagents (see above). It is not necessary to sterilize tips and tubes for PCR work.

(g) Screw-capped tubes are more suitable for storage of extracted DNA and RNA as opening snap-on lids can lead to aerosol formation, and because the operator's glove may come into contact with the underside of the lid.

(h) All equipment should be decontaminated immediately if it comes into contact with solutions containing viral nucleic acids, and at regular intervals during normal use of the laboratory. HCl (1 M) rapidly destroys DNA and is a good decontaminant for non-metallic items. Glutaraldehyde and hypochlorite solutions may also be used but are less effective at removing DNA; only the former should be used for metal items.

2.1.3 PCR room

Ideally, the PCR should be carried out in a separate room from both the sample preparation and 'clean' areas. As this may not always be possible, the reactions can be set up on a designated bench in the sample preparation room.

i. Equipment

The following equipment should be reserved for this stage of the procedure:

- dedicated $-20\,°C$ and $-70\,°C$ freezers for storage of clinical samples, extracted DNA and extracted RNA
- one or more programmable thermal cyclers
- complete set of pipettes, supply of pipette tips and tubes for PCR

ii. Precautions

(a) Buffers for PCR and/or RT steps should be prepared, in advance, in the 'clean' room.

(b) The PCR/RT reactions should be set up on a use-once bench cover.

(c) Positive controls should contain only low amounts of target DNA or RNA, to avoid contamination of other tubes in the PCR, and to act as a 'realistic' guide to the performance of the PCR (see Section 4.2).

(d) After amplification, the tubes should be immediately removed from the laboratory and stored in a freezer separate from non-amplified samples and PCR reagents.

2.1.4 General laboratory

A major cause of contamination of PCRs is previously amplified DNA. Therefore, a separate laboratory is required for setting up 'second' PCRs (if nested primers are used), agarose or polyacrylamide gel electrophoresis of PCR products, facilities for viewing and photographing ethidium bromide stained gels, carrying out restriction digests, sequencing reactions, and so on. It must be assumed that all items of equipment, all buffers, laboratory coats, and all disposables that have been in this laboratory are irreversibly contaminated with viral DNA. Therefore, it is imperative that nothing should be taken from this laboratory back into the PCR, sample preparation, or 'clean' rooms. For example, empty tip racks from this laboratory should not be refilled in the clean room. Laboratory coats for the different areas must be kept separate, and gloves removed and hands washed when moving between rooms. It helps if the rooms reserved for PCR use are some distance away from the general laboratory.

The steps outlined above to avoid contamination have so far proved successful in our laboratory. However, other groups working regularly with PCR have had to go to extreme lengths to prevent contamination, such as wearing caps and face masks when extracting samples and showering before setting up PCRs. Obviously, some laboratories have greater problems than others; in particular, research laboratories that are currently, or were in the past, producing or using recombinant viral sequences will have a far worse problem than laboratories that are embarking on DNA detection methods for the first time (see Section 4.2.3, point (a)).

2.2 Sample handling

The following sections outline tested methods for preparing clinical specimens for DNA and RNA extraction.

2.2.1 Extraction of viruses from plasma or cerebrospinal fluid

Free or immune-complexed virions in plasma or cerebrospinal fluid (CSF) may be unstable. For example, the amount of hepatitis C virus (HCV) RNA recoverable from plasma can decline as much as 10-fold if the sample is stored overnight at 4 °C. In our laboratory, all routine samples are divided on arrival, with one half being kept at 4 °C for routine HBV, HCV, and HIV serology, and the other half immediately frozen should it prove necessary to carry out PCR at a later stage. In many circumstances (e.g. to enhance sensitivity of detection), it is desirable to enrich the sample for virus prior to extraction. Methods for precipitation of HCV and HBV from plasma by polyethylene glycol have been described (21). Alternatively, virus can be pelleted from plasma or CSF (diluted in PBS to make up the tube volume) in a Beckman SW50.1 rotor (capacity 6 × 5 ml) at 40 000 r.p.m. or a Sorvall SH-80 rotor (capacity 8 × 10 ml) at 28 000 r.p.m for 1–2 h prior to extraction by either the Proteinase K or RNAzol methods (*Protocols 1* and *2*).

2.2.2 Peripheral blood mononuclear cells

Peripheral blood mononuclear cells (PBMCs) can be separated from whole, fresh, anti-coagulated blood by layering on to an equal volume of a lymphocyte separating medium (e.g. Nycoprep from Nycomed), and centrifugation at 900 g for 30 min at room temperature. PBMCs collecting at the interface between the upper, plasma layer and the Ficoll are then harvested, washed and pelleted in PBS by further centrifugation prior to DNA or RNA extraction.

2.2.3 Cells from swabs

These should be dispersed in transport medium or PBS and pelleted by low-speed centrifugation prior to DNA or RNA extraction (*Protocols 1* and *2*).

2.2.4 Pieces of tissue sent to the virology laboratory

These should be dissected into small pieces ($\leq 1\,\text{mm}^3$) with a new razor blade in a Petri dish on ice. The cellular material should then be immediately transferred to lysis buffer (*Protocol 1*) or RNAzol solution (*Protocol 2*) for extraction of viral nucleic acids. Specimens should be processed quickly to avoid degradation of viral nucleic acids by autolysis. A separate blade and Petri dish should be used for each sample to minimize contamination.

2.2.5 Non-immune complexed viruses

Antibody attached to a solid phase can be used to extract viral particles from clinical specimens prior to DNA or RNA extraction (22–24).

2.3 DNA extraction

The ideal substrate for the PCR is chemically pure DNA and, to this end, a number of protocols have been developed to extract DNA from cells, plasma, and other types of clinical specimens. The choice of method is inevitably a compromise between purity of DNA and the amount of time available for extraction of often large numbers of samples. There has been considerable interest in devising methods for preparation of amplifiable DNA with the minimum numbers of steps and lowest risk of contamination by exogenous DNA. The following protocol has been used extensively by the author and others in the department, and represents a reasonable compromise between quality of DNA and ease of use, yielding fairly pure, high molecular weight DNA, which can be stored indefinitely at $-20\,°\text{C}$ without obvious degradation. Methods which do not use phenol/chloroform extraction yield DNA with variable amounts of inhibitors and nucleases that interfere with amplification and prevent long-term storage. In the opinion of the author, the extra time spent in extracting DNA by the supplied protocol compared with simpler methods will be amply repaid by the gain in sensitivity and reproducibility of the PCR. In the future, however, if the PCR is to be used widely, simpler protocols will need to be developed that do not interfere with the sensitivity and specificity of the amplification reaction. Methods that extract DNA or RNA directly from treated clinical specimens by adsorption (25, 26), filtration, or inactivation of nucleases prior to amplification (17, 27–30) are possible alternatives to the traditional methods of nucleic acid extraction, and require critical evaluation with standardized reagents.

Protocol 1. Extraction of DNA

Reagents

- Lysis buffer (50 mM Tris–HCl (pH 8.0), 50 mM EDTA (pH 8.0), 100 mM NaCl, (0.0001% (w/v) herring sperm DNA (Boehringer), if DNA is extracted from plasma or CSF)
- 1% w/v Proteinase K (Sigma) in distilled H_2O ($\times$ 100 stock)

- 10% *N*-lauroylsarcosine ('Sarkosyl', BDH)
- Phenol (water-saturated; Rathburn)
- Chloroform
- Chilled 100% ethanol

Method

1. Resuspend virus pellet or up to 5×10^6 cells in 0.4 ml of lysis buffer, premixed with 4.4 µl Proteinase K stock solution, on ice.

2. Add 44 µl of *N*-lauroylsarcosine (to give a final concentration of 1%); mix well.

3. Incubate for 2 h at 65 °C in a hot block.

4. Extract with equal volumes of phenol (once or twice) and chloroform (once).

5. Add two volumes of ethanol; mix well; leave for 2 h at −20 °C.

6. Centrifuge tube for 15 min at 10 000 *g* at 4 °C.

7. Remove ethanol solution carefully; dry DNA pellet at 50 °C for 10–15 min.

8. Resuspend in 20–200 µl of distilled water (to ensure adequate solubilization), incubate sample at 50 °C for 15–30 min with frequent vortex mixing.

9. Assess DNA concentration and purity by spectrophotometry at 260 and 280 nm.

2.4 Handling and extracting RNA

Unlike DNA, RNA is highly susceptible to degradation by trace quantities of nucleases found in the general environment. The following section lists some general precautions that need to be taken to prevent loss of RNA during handling in the laboratory. Further details can be obtained from general laboratory manuals (31, 32).

2.4.1 Precautions

(a) Always wear gloves when handling or dispensing solutions used for RNA extraction or reverse transcription. Quite apart from contributing to operator safety, gloves reduce contamination by skin and skin flakes which are a particularly rich source of nucleases.

(b) Avoid using glassware for the storage of solutions used for RNA work.

(c) Unused plasticware can be assumed to be free of nucleases. However, care should be taken when handling tips and tubes to avoid contact with skin, clothing, or bench-covers when handling. Bags of tips and tubes should be kept sealed when not in use.

(d) Chemicals used to prepare buffers should be weighed out into plastic containers with a flamed spatula.

(e) To prepare nuclease-free water and buffers, add 0.05 (w/v) diethylpyrocarbonate (DEPC) and autoclave at 121 °C for 30 min after 2–24 h. Note that DEPC cannot be used to treat solutions containing amide groups (e.g. Tris). Care should be taken to avoid using autoclaves that are contaminated with viral DNA (see Section 2.1.1).

(f) Some suppliers of reverse transcriptase include 10 × RT buffer for cDNA synthesis, which can be used in place of the RT buffer described in *Protocol 2*.

(g) Solutions can be supplemented with nuclease inhibitors such as RNAsin (see *Protocol 3*) or vanadyl-ribonucleoside complexes.

(h) Molecular biology grade nucleotide triphosphates, DMSO, and the virus-specific primers used in the RT reaction have worked satisfactorily in the protocols listed below without anti-nuclease treatment.

2.4.2 Extraction of RNA

Successful extraction of RNA from clinical specimens requires considerably more care than DNA extraction since RNA is highly susceptible to degradation by intracellular nucleases *in vivo*, and *in vitro* by nucleases that appear to be ubiquitous in the environment. Furthermore, for detection by PCR, it has first to be reverse transcribed into DNA by enzymes that are generally less tolerant of impurities than *Taq* polymerase. The following protocol (33), adapted from a well established extraction method for cellular RNA (34), is relatively quick and easy to carry out on large numbers and different types of virological specimens.

Protocol 2. Extraction of RNA

Reagents

- Denaturing solution (4 M guanidinium thiocyanate, 25 mM sodium citrate (pH 7.0); 1% (w/v) N-lauroylsarcosine)
- 2-Mercaptoethanol
- 2 M sodium acetate
- Phenol (water-saturated; Rathburn)
- Chloroform
- Chilled isopropanol
- Carrier tRNA (if extracting RNA from plasma or CSF)

Method

1. Immediately before use, pre-mix the following for each sample:
   - 0.5 ml denaturing solution

121

Protocol 1. *Continued*

- 3.65 μl 2-mercaptoethanol
- 50 μl sodium acetate solution
- 0.5 ml phenol

The presence of guanidinium thiocyanate ensures that phenol will mix fully with the aqueous phase.

2. Add 1 ml of this solution to virus or cell pellet on ice; mix to ensure complete dissolution.

3. Add 100 μl of chloroform and incubate on ice for 5–15 min with frequent mixing.

4. Centrifuge at 10 000 g at 4 °C for 15 min in a refrigerated microcentrifuge.

5. Carefully remove upper aqueous layer by aspiration, avoiding any material at the interface, and transfer to a new tube.

6. Extract once with an equal volume of chloroform (if upper phase remains cloudy after spinning, go back to step 5).

7. Add equal volume of chilled isopropanol (approximately 600 μl); mix well and leave at − 20 °C for at least 2 h to precipitate RNA.

8. Spin tube at 10 000 g at 4 °C for 15 min, after which a minute pellet of RNA may be seen at the bottom of the tube.

9. Carefully remove the supernatant by aspiration (it may be desirable to wash the RNA in ice-cold 70 % ethanol, followed by centrifugation for 10 min).

10. Dry pellet at 50 °C for 10–15 min.

11. Dissolve in 20 μl of nuclease-free water.

12. Run a portion of the extracted RNA on an agarose gel, pre-stained with ethidium bromide (*Protocol 6*) to measure concentration of RNA and degree of degradation after extraction (28S, 18S, and 5S bands of rRNA can be easily resolved in RNA extracted from mammalian cells if this method is followed correctly).

3. Amplification reactions

3.1 Reverse transcription of RNA

The following method (*Protocol 3*) has proved highly reliable for the detection of HIV and HCV RNA extracted from plasma by *Protocol 2*, using a wide range of different primer combinations. For double-stranded RNA viruses, it will be necessary to denature the RNA before adding the reverse transcriptase (e.g. references 18, 35, 36). The method described here uses a virus-specific primer for initiation of cDNA synthesis from the viral RNA.

Other investigators have used random priming with hexameric oligonucleo-tides; the author is not aware of any studies that formally compare the effectiveness of the two methods. The efficiency of detection of RNA is critically dependent on the spacing of the primers used subsequently in the PCR (33), because the size distribution of reverse transcripts is such that only a minority exceed 1000 bases in length. Thus the wider the spacing of primers, the fewer transcripts will be long enough to be amplifiable in the PCR (see Section 4.5.2 on quantification of viral RNA sequences).

In some circumstances, it may be necessary to detect specifically viral mRNA or genomic RNA in the presence of viral DNA of the same sequence (i.e. to study virus expression of a normally latent DNA virus, or to dis-tinguish viral and proviral forms of retroviruses). Such samples require pre-treatment with DNase. Although such methods have been widely used, it is difficult to obtain DNase that is completely free of RNase activity; furthermore, DNA that is complexed with protein is resistant to digestion by DNase. The reader is referred to a published protocol for practical informa-tion (33).

Protocol 3. Reverse transcription[a]

Reagents

- Reverse transcription (RT) buffer (10×:500 mM Tris–HCl (pH 8.0), 500 mM KCl, 50 mM MgCl$_2$, 50 mM DTT, 0.5% (w/v) RNase-free bovine serum albumin (Boehringer, cat. no. 711454) in nuclease-free water)
- Nucleoside triphosphates (Boehringer, 10 mM each of dATP (cat. no. 1051440), dCTP (cat. no. 1051458), dGTP (cat. no.

1051466), and TTP (cat. no. 1051482) in nuclease-free water)
- Dimethyl sulphoxide
- RNAsin (Boehringer or Promega)
- Reverse transcriptase (from avian myelo-blastosis virus; *c.* 10 U/µl; Boehringer or Promega)

Method

1. Mix together the following reagents in an ice bath in the stated order:
   - 7.5 µl of RNase-free water
   - 3 µl of dimethyl sulphoxide
   - 100 ng of virus-specific primer (in 1 µl)
   - 2 µl 10 × RT buffer
   - 2 µl of nucleoside triphosphate mixture
   - 0.5 µl of RNAsin
   - 3 µl of RNA, prepared according to *Protocol 2*
   - 1 µl of reverse transcriptase

2. Mix contents of tube; incubate for 30–60 min at 42 °C.

3. Pulse spin tube; add to PCR (*Protocol 4*).

Protocol 3. *Continued*

4. Alternatively, store at −20 °C until required; note, however, that in practice, cDNA produced in this reaction appears to be slightly unstable. Long-term storage leads to significant reductions in the amount of target DNA amplifiable by the PCR.

---

[a] This protocol was kindly contributed by L. Q. Zhang (33), Institute of Cell, Animal, and Population Biology, University of Edinburgh for the detection of HIV RNA in plasma.

3.2 Amplification of DNA

The following buffers and temperatures (*Protocol 4*) are suitable for the majority of primer/template combinations. The degree of optimization of the reaction conditions, in terms of both buffer composition and temperatures, depends critically on the specific application. As will be described in Section 4, the gain in specificity and sensitivity of nested PCR methods, particularly those with narrow primer spacings, considerably reduces the requirement for optimization of the reaction, as the method is capable of detecting single molecules of target DNA in fairly adverse conditions. However, methods that use single pairs of primers are less sensitive, have limited specificity due to co-amplification of non-target DNA, and are thus more critically dependent on the precise amplification conditions used. Some suggestions on how PCR conditions may be optimized are given in Section 4.1.2.

Protocol 4. Amplification of DNA

Equipment and reagents

- PCR buffer (10×: 200 mM Tris–HCl (pH 8.8), 500 mM KCl, 15 mM $MgCl_2$, 0.5% Triton X-100)
- Nucleoside triphosphates (100 × stock; 3 mM each of dATP, dCTP, dGTP, and dTTP)
- 15–60 μM sense primer[a] (for a 20-mer, 100–400 μg/ml)
- 15–60 μM antisense primer[a]
- Mineral oil (BDH, cat. no. 29436)
- *Taq* polymerase (Cetus, Promega, Northumbria, Biologicals, or Boehringer)
- Programmable thermal cycler (e.g. Techne PHC-1 or PHC-2, Perkin Elmer thermal cycler, or Hybaid thermal reactor)

Method

1. For each sample, pre-mix:
   - 5 μl of 10 × PCR buffer
   - 38 μl of water
   - 0.5 μl of nucleoside triphosphate mixture
   - 0.25 μl of sense primer (approximately 4–16 pmol)[b]
   - 0.25 μl of antisense primer

- 1 unit of *Taq* polymerase (0.1–0.25 µl at most manufacturers' supplied concentrations)
- 5 µl of DNA or cDNA sample[c]

For amplifying multiple samples, it is easier to make up a stock containing all but the sample, and adding 45 µl to each tube. Cover with a drop of mineral oil.

2. Transfer immediately to a thermal cycler set with the following temperatures and times:
   - (a) 94 °C, 35 sec
   - (b) 50 °C, 40 sec
   - (c) 68 °C, 150 sec

3. Samples should be amplified over 25–35 cycles (25 cycles is sufficient with outer and inner primers in nested PCR protocols).

4. The samples should be heated at 68–72 °C for 5 min at the end of the last cycle to terminate uncompleted strands.

5. Amplified DNA is stable, and can be stored at 4 °C (or at −20 °C long-term) before analysis by Southern/dot blotting (*Protocol 5*) or nested PCR (*Protocol 6*).

[a] Primers are available from several commercial and academic institutions in many countries. For example, primers can be ordered by post, fax, or telephone at a cost of £3.50 per base (0.2 µM scale) from Oswel DNA Service, Department of Chemistry, University of Edinburgh, West Mains Road, Edinburgh EH9 3JJ, UK (Tel. 31 650 4792; Fax. 31 662 4054).

[b] Although the precise concentration of primers normally matters little in the range given above, it is recommended that approximately equal amounts of sense and antisense primers are added.

[c] For the reasons outlined in Section 1.2, do not add more than 5 µl of cDNA (from Protocol 3), or more than 2 µg of DNA (from *Protocol 1*). Increase the volume of PCR (up to 200 µl) if amplification of larger amounts is required. Adjust the volume of water added to allow for different sample volumes.

4. Detection of amplified product

4.1 Overview of methods

This section gives detailed protocols for two straightforward and tested methods for detection of amplified DNA. For the reasons discussed in Section 1.2, the degree of amplification possible with a single pair of primers is often limited to around 10^6–10^7 times the starting amount, irrespective of the number of 'doubling' cycles employed. Thus the amount of PCR product obtained from the amplification of small amounts of target DNA may be extremely limited. Furthermore, there may be variable amounts of amplified non-viral DNA in the PCR product that prevent identification of specific DNA.

The size of amplified DNA can be predicted from the spacing of the primers used in the amplification reaction (*Figure 1*), and simple agarose gel electrophoresis of the PCR product with staining by ethidium bromide may reveal a band of DNA of the appropriate mobility. The method requires that at least 1–10 ng of DNA is produced by the PCR. Although the size of the amplified DNA may serve to distinguish it from non-specifically amplified DNA, this may be difficult in situations where numerous hybrid bands are produced, of which one may, by chance, happen to be of the same size as the amplified viral DNA.

4.2 Controls for PCR

Every time the PCR is used to detect viral sequences in clinical specimens, it is essential to include a number of controls to ensure that the assay is performing satisfactorily, in terms of sensitivity, specificity, and avoidance of contamination by exogenous DNA sequences.

4.2.1 Positive controls

Positive controls should be used at each stage of the PCR, to ensure that each is working adequately. Thus, during extraction of DNA or RNA from a clinical specimen, one should always repeat the extraction of a known positive clinical sample. After extraction of RNA, a known positive RNA sample should be added in as a control for the cDNA synthesis reaction. A positive DNA or cDNA sample should then be used in the PCR. Finally, a known positive PCR product should be included in each of the two detection methods described below (*Protocols 5* and *6*). Positive results from all three controls (or four in RNA PCR) will thus validate the assay. Negative results from one, two, or three of the controls will indicate at which stage the assay went wrong. It should be stressed that the minimum amount of target DNA necessary to give a positive result should be used. Positive controls with large amounts of DNA do not give a realistic guide to the performance of the assay, and they are more liable to contaminate other samples.

4.2.2 Negative controls

It is recommended that negative controls are also included at each stage in the PCR. Ideally, the negative control for the DNA or RNA extraction stage should be a known negative clinical specimen of the type being extracted. For many situations the reader should consider the ethical position before using samples from other laboratory workers as controls for PCR. As for positive controls, negative RNA, negative DNA or cDNA, and finally negative PCR product should be added in during the assay and analysed with the clinical specimens. These controls provide a comprehensive check for contamination, and can indicate precisely where it occurred.

4.2.3 False–positive results from contamination

Contamination in the PCR laboratory may arise from three different sources:

(a) Many diagnostic/research laboratories use or have used hybridization methods for virological detection, such as *in situ* or Southern blotting. Such procedures necessitate the use of relatively large amounts of recombinant viral DNA for use as probes. It is almost inevitable that such methods will cause contamination of the equipment and laboratory space used for such methods, as well as of departmental distilled water supplies, chemicals, autoclaves, and so on. In such cases, it is essential that the rooms designated for PCR work should be in parts of the department that have never been used for such work, and that all reagents for sample extraction and PCR be re-ordered.

(b) The majority of clinical specimens contain very little viral DNA. However, some viruses may occasionally be present at very high titre (e.g. certain carriers of hepatitis B surface antigen, particularly those positive for hepatitis B e antigen, individuals with recent B19 parvovirus infection, vesicle fluid in herpes simplex or zoster infection, and adenovirus in faecal specimens), and careless extraction of DNA may lead to contamination of other samples, pipettes, solutions used for DNA extraction, and the containment hood.

(c) Vials with PCR product can often contain extremely large amounts of DNA that may lead to contamination of subsequent amplification reactions. This type of contamination is progressive, in that it occurs with increasing frequency the more the PCR with a particular set of primers is used. The steps outlined in Section 2.1 to separate physically the preparation of reagents and samples from areas where DNA is electrophoresed are the most important preventative measure.

The nested PCR (*Protocol 6*) is much less prone to contamination than single PCRs (*Protocol 5*), because the product DNA from the second reaction cannot contaminate the first PCR, while contamination of the second reaction is of no consequence as it cannot be detected by agarose gel electrophoresis of the final product. Thus, provided the first PCR product is handled carefully (e.g. by pulse spinning it before opening, and storing it separately from clinical specimens and PCR reagents), very few problems from this type of contamination will occur.

Although prevention is better than cure, two methods that modify amplified DNA to reduce the problem of contamination of samples have been described. The first method uses dUTP in place of dTTP in the PCR buffer (37). The 'DNA' produced in these modified conditions differs from ordinary DNA in its susceptibility to degradation by uracil-*N*-glycosidase, and pre-incubation of PCR samples in this enzyme prior to heat-cycling will eliminate contaminating 'DNA' that may be present, at the expense of possibly reduced efficiency of amplification and the risk of incomplete denaturation of the enzyme during early cycles of the PCR. The other approach is to supplement the PCR buffer with the psoralen derivative 4'-AMDMIP (38). Product DNA can be cross-linked and rendered non-copyable by exposing the reaction tube to ultraviolet light after amplification. However, 4'-AMDMIP may reduce the efficiency of amplification, the cross-linked DNA will be more difficult to detect by hybridization, and cannot be used in nested PCR protocols.

4.3 Hybridization

Positive identification of amplified viral DNA can be achieved by hybridization. In such methods, product DNA is denatured in alkali, blotted on to a nylon filter (Southern or dot blotting; see Chapter 3), and hybridized with a labelled oligonucleotide 'probe' that is complementary to part of the target viral DNA sequence (but excluding the primer sequences). After washing of the nylon filter to remove non-hybridized probe, target DNA can be detected by autoradiography (if the probe was radiolabelled) or further incubations with conjugate and substrate (if the probe was biotin- or digoxygenin-labelled). This hybridization method will permit the specific identification of amplified bands containing the viral sequence; hybrid product, ultimately derived from non-viral sequences, will not be labelled. Furthermore, hybridization is several orders of magnitude more sensitive than ethidium bromide staining. The combination of specificity and sensitivity achieved by hybridization has led to the development of several gel-based and non-gel-based (e.g. dot/slot blotting) detection methods for amplified DNA (8, 29, 39–44; also see Chapter 3). It is beyond the scope of this chapter to evaluate each one; however, a straightforward and tested method for PCR product detection by Southern and dot blotting is given in *Protocol 5*.

4.3.1 Hybridization conditions

Although probes can be made from cloned DNA sequences corresponding to the amplified sequences, most investigators have used chemically synthesized oligonucleotide probes for hybridization. Such probes vary both in length (20–50 nucleotides) and in G+C content, both of which affect the 'melting' temperature (T_m, i.e. the maximum temperature at which the oligonucleotide just remains hybridized) and thus the conditions under which the hybridization is carried out. The following relation (45, 46) allows the calculation of the T_m for oligonucleotide probes likely to be used for hybridization (lengths ranging from 20–50 bases):

$$T_m = 81 + 16.6 \, (\log_{10}[Na^+]) + 0.4 \, (\%[G+C]) - 600/n - 1.5(\% \text{ mismatch})$$

where $[Na^+]$ is the molarity of sodium ions in the hybridization buffer, $\%[G+C]$ the G+C content of the primer, and n the length of the primer. The effect of mismatches on the T_m depends on the type of mismatch (e.g. pyrimidine–pyrimidine pairs are more disruptive to base pairing than purine–

purine ones), and where they occur in the duplex. The figure of $1.5\,°C/\%$ mismatch used in the formula (46) is therefore only an approximation. As an example, the T_m of a 20 base oligonucleotide with a 45% G+C content in the hybridization buffer described in *Protocol 5* ($6 \times$ SSC, 2% SDS $\equiv 900 + 90 + 70\,mM\ Na^+$ ions), with one mismatch is $81 + (16.6 \times 0.025) + (0.4 \times 45) - (600/20) - (1.5 \times 5) = 62\,°C$.

Temperatures approximately $10\text{--}15\,°C$ below the calculated T_m are normally suitable for the hybridization and washing steps described in *Protocol 5*. However, this temperature can be increased by $5\text{--}10\,°C$ to reduce non-specific binding if this is a problem, and lowered if weak or absent hybridization signals are obtained.

Protocol 5. Detection of amplified DNA by hybridization [a,b]

Equipment and reagents

(a) Southern blotting:
- Agarose
- 10 × stock TBE buffer (0.89 M Tris, 0.89 M boric acid, 0.02 M EDTA (pH 8.0))
- 10 × gel loading buffer (25% Ficoll, 0.25% bromophenol blue in water)

(b) Southern and dot blotting:
- Denaturing solution (0.5 M NaOH, 1.5 M NaCl)
- Neutralizing solution (1 M ammonium acetate, 0.02 M NaOH)
- Nylon (e.g. Hybond-N, Amersham, cat. no. RPN303N) or nitrocellulose filter
- Oligonucleotide complementary to part of amplified sequence

- [γ-^{32}P]ATP (*c.* 3000 Ci/mmol, Amersham, cat. no. PB10168)
- Kinase buffer (500 mM Tris–HCl (pH 7.6), 100 mM MgCl$_2$, 50 mM DTT, 1 mM spermidine, 1 mM EDTA (pH 8.0))
- T4 polynucleotide kinase (5 U/μl, Boehringer, cat. no. 174645)
- Denhardt's solution (2% BSA-Pentax Fraction V (Boehringer cat. no. 735086), 2% Ficoll, 2% polyvinylpyrollidone)
- 20 × SSC (3 M NaCl, 0.3 M sodium citrate, adjusted to pH 7.0 with NaOH)
- X-ray film (X-Omat R, Kodak)
- Light-tight cassette (optionally with intensifying screens to increase signal).

Method

A. *Southern blotting*

1. Mix PCR product with 0.1 volume of gel loading buffer.

2. Electrophorese on 1.0% agarose gel in 1 × TBE, using 1 × TBE electrophoresis buffer at 2.5 V/cm. Continue until the blue dye front has migrated $10\text{--}20\,cm$.

3. Immerse gel in two 500 ml changes of denaturing solution for 15 min each, with gentle rocking.

4. Neutralize in two 500 ml changes of neutralizing solution for 20 min each with gentle rocking.

5. Place gel on clean glass plate, and overlay with a sheet of nylon filter (**important: nylon filters must not be handled without gloves**), three sheets of filter paper soaked in neutralizing solution, five sheets of dry paper, and a stack of paper towels. Finally add a glass plate, and place a

Protocol 5. *Continued*

2 kg weight on top. Allow blotting of DNA from the gel to the nylon filter for 1–2 h.

6. Recover filter, and wash for 2 min in 200 ml 2 × SSC.

7. Place nylon filter face down on Saran wrap (cling film), and place on UV transilluminator for 5 min to fix DNA to filter (nitrocellulose filters should be baked at 80 °C for 2 h to fix DNA).

B. *Dot blotting*

1. Mix 5–10 µl of PCR product with 100 µl of denaturing solution.

2. Incubate at room temperature for 10 min.

3. Add entire sample to well in a dot or slot blot manifold (manufacturers include Bio-Rad). Draw sample through under vacuum.

4. Draw through a further 500 µl of 2 × SSC.

5. Recover filter from apparatus, continue as for Southern blotting, steps 6 and 7.

6. Alternatively, 2–3 µl volumes of PCR product can be mixed with 1 µl of 2 M NaOH, 1.5 M NaCl, and directly spotted on to a sheet of nylon filter. Continue as for Southern blotting, steps 6 and 7.

C. *Probe labelling*

End-labelling of oligonucleotides (produces sufficient for one hybridization reaction; can be re-used):

1. Mix together 11.5 µl of water, 8 pmol (in 1 µl) of oligonucleotide, 2 µl of kinase buffer, 3.5 µl of [γ-^{32}P]dATP (approximately 35 µCi, depending on activity date) and 2 µl of T4 polynucleotide kinase.

2. Incubate for 1 h at 37 °C.

3. Incubate at 65 °C for 10 min to heat-inactivate the kinase.

D. *Hybridization*

1. To prepare prehybridization/hybridization solution, mix together:
   - 2.5 ml of Denhardt's solution
   - 5 ml of 20% (w/v) SDS solution in water
   - 15 ml 20 × SSC
   - 27.5 ml of water

2. Seal filter between two polythene sheets with a bag sealer, together with prehybridization solution (use approximately 30 ml for a 20 × 20 cm nylon filter).

3. Incubate at 50 °C for 10 min to 1 h taped down on a rotary shaker (100 r.p.m.).

4. Recover filter, reseal in new bag together with 20 ml of hybridization solution containing probe prepared above. **Caution: take care to avoid spillage of ^{32}P label; double seal hybridization bag**.

5. Incubate for 1–18 h at 50 °C [c] as described in step 3.

6. Recover filter, and wash successively in three changes of 100 ml volumes of 6 × SSC at 50 °C for 30 min each. The washing solutions and dish should be pre-warmed to 50 °C before use. Increase the washing temperature by 5–10 °C if a high background is obtained.

7. Wrap nylon filter in Saran wrap, expose to X-ray film in cassette with intensifying screens for 2–72 h depending on strength of signal. If using intensifying screens, expose film to filter at −70 °C to increase sensitivity and resolution.

[a] This protocol was kindly supplied by Dr S. W. Chan, Department of Medical Microbiology, University of Edinburgh.

[b] All steps described here should be carried out in the general laboratory to avoid contamination of PCR samples and reagents. It is assumed that the operator is familiar with the regulations concerning the safe handling and disposal of radiolabel, and that the laboratory is equipped and approved for use of [32]P.

[c] The temperatures and washing solutions given here should be suitable for use with oligonucleotide probes that are around 20–25 base pairs long. See Section 4.3.1 to calculate the T_m for probes of different lengths and G+C contents. A hybridization temperature 10–15 °C below the T_m is recommended for initial experiments.

4.4 Evaluation of the performance of the PCR

It is strongly recommended that the sensitivity and reproducibility of the PCR is measured in an objective way before using it for diagnostic purposes. This will enable an assessment of its performance (PCR methods using hybridization as a means of detecting amplified product can often detect as few as 5–20 copies of target DNA (30, 40, 41, 43, 44, 47–50) and will give some idea of what 'positive' and 'negative' results with clinical specimens actually mean. The best source of standard DNA for quantification purposes is purified recombinant DNA that has been accurately quantified by spectrophotometry. However, this may not always be readily available, and an alternative is to use PCR product itself, as follows:

(a) Amplify a known positive DNA sample.

(b) Run half of the sample on a pre-stained agarose gel (*Protocol 6*), along with a series of dilutions of a standard size marker (e.g. pBR322 digested with *Hae*III, amounts ranging from 200 ng to 10 ng).

(c) Compare the fluorescent intensity of the amplified DNA with each dilution of a band in the size marker that most closely matches the size of the PCR product. The amount of DNA in each band of the marker DNA is in direct proportion to its size.

(d) Excise the PCR product band from gel and place in tube. Weigh tube to estimate the volume of agarose.

(e) Warm tube to 37 °C to melt agarose; dilute in 100 volumes of pre-warmed TE buffer to disperse agarose, assuming a density of 1 g/ml.

The number of molecules of either the recombinant or PCR-amplified DNA can be calculated as follows:

$$\text{No. of molecules} = \frac{[\text{DNA}] \times 10^{-9} \times A}{m \times l}$$

where [DNA] refers to the amount of DNA in ng, A is Avogadro's number, *m* the average molecular weight of a base pair, and *l* the length of the PCR product (see Section 1.2). For example, 10 ng of a 500 bp PCR product contains approximately 2×10^{10} copies of target DNA. If this band was excised from the agarose gel in a block weighing 0.5 g, and diluted into 50 ml (see above), then the final concentration of DNA would be 4×10^8 copies/ml. This DNA should now be diluted to a final concentration of around 2×10^6 copies/ml in a 200 µg/ml solution of herring sperm DNA. This DNA can now be used relatively safely as a positive control for PCRs (**do not bring more concentrated DNA into the PCR room**). To investigate the sensitivity of the PCR, it is suggested that 10 000, 1000, 100, 10, 1, and 0 copies of target DNA are amplified in replicate by *Protocol 5*. The PCR is working satisfactorily if 100 copies can be detected by Southern blot or dot hybridization. If not, it may be necessary to vary the reaction conditions of the PCR to obtain optimal amplification of DNA, while avoiding non-specific amplification of non-target DNA.

4.4.1 Optimization of the PCR

(a) The sensitivity and specificity of the PCR is greatly influenced by the concentration of Mg^{2+} ions. Too high a concentration of $MgCl_2$ in the PCR buffer may promote non-specific amplification, while too low a concentration will reduce the rate at which target DNA is copied. The optimum concentration of $MgCl_2$ depends on the primers used, other components in the PCR buffer, and the amount of non-target DNA in the reaction. Thus, it is normally necessary to optimize this parameter during the development of the PCR. Concentrations in the range 0.5–8 mM are recommended for initial titrations. Under some circumstances the concentration of *Taq* polymerase, nucleotide triphosphates, and primers can also influence the specificity and efficiency of the amplification reaction. Note that the optimum concentration of Mg^{2+} is altered to a certain extent by the concentration of these other components of the PCR.

(b) The composition of PCR buffers varies widely between published methods. Some include protein (such as albumin or gelatin) instead of, or in addition to, a non-ionic detergent. Although there have been few studies that formally compare the effect that these additives have on amplification, it may be worth trying alternatives if the steps taken to optimize the PCR are unsuccessful.

(c) The optimum temperature for hybridization of the primers to target DNA should be used. This temperature is a function of the length and base composition of the primers (the longer the primer, and the higher the G+C content, the higher the annealing temperature). The T_m of the primer is influenced by the concentration of the different components in the PCR buffer; in particular the presence of Mg^{2+} ions enhances duplex formation, and invalidates the simple formula for T_m given in Section 4.3.1. However, a commonly used rule-of-thumb is to add on 4°C for every G or C residue in the primer sequence, and 2°C for every A or T. Thus, a 20-mer with a 45% G+C content should have a T_m of very approximately 58°C, and 54°C if one of the G or C residues is mismatched. As with Southern and dot blotting, the annealing temperature should be substantially below the T_m to promote efficient hybridization. Thus the temperature of 50°C recommended as a starting point in *Protocol 4* should be suitable for primers 18–24 base pairs long. **It is important for optimization that the T_m of the two primers used in the PCR should be within 5°C of each other.**

(d) The temperatures and times given for primer extension (68°C) and denaturation (94°C) should normally be suitable for all primers with spacings of less than 500 base pairs, and should not need to be varied. However, PCR with wider primer spacings requires increases in the concentration of nucleotide triphosphates and in extension and denaturation times.

(e) Different primers will amplify human or other non-target sequences to varying extents. Some primers may be unusable for this reason; if excessive non-specific DNA is produced during the PCR, and the steps taken to remedy this are ineffective, it may be necessary to obtain a different set of primers.

(f) PCRs rarely benefit from increased numbers of cycles, as they promote the copying of non-target DNA. Little effective amplification can be achieved by increasing the number over 40.

4.4.2 Quantification by PCR

It is beyond the scope of this chapter to discuss the different protocols that have been developed to quantify target DNA by amplification and hybridization. Most methods so far described use the amount of product as an indication of how much target DNA there was in the original material (51–57). This method is subject to two major constraints. Firstly, the PCR is saturated by large amounts (> 100 ng) of product DNA, so quantitative measurements can only be usefully made over a relatively narrow range of target DNA concentrations. Secondly, the rate at which target DNA accumulates is highly variable, and depends critically on the precise reaction conditions and on the amount of non-target DNA present in the reaction, each of which can vary between assay runs. To overcome this latter problem, most quantification methods co-amplify a limiting amount of control DNA with a second set of primers in the reaction mixture (53, 56, 58). Thus, the amount of specific product can be related to the amount of amplified control DNA, assuming that variation in the assay conditions affects the rate of amplification of both sequences equally. Equal rates of amplification can be assured if the control

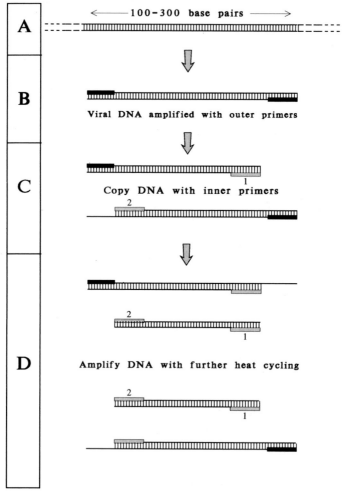

Figure 2. PCR with nested primers. (A) Viral DNA. (B) Amplification with outer primers (solid boxes) as in *Figure 1* to generate 100–300 base pair fragment. (C) product DNA denatured and copied from inner primers (hatched boxes) in first cycle. (D) Second cycle of PCR generating four copies of product DNA. PCR was continued for 25 cycles.

DNA is the same viral sequence as the DNA being quantified, apart from a single extra restriction site, which allows the two amplified species to be differentiated after amplification (59). The papers cited above should be referred to for practical information on quantitative PCR.

4.5 Nested PCR

The second method for detection of amplified DNA is to use the PCR itself, for a second time (4, 12, 21, 27, 60–62). As explained in Section 1.2, the formation of hybrid DNA may limit the amount of amplification achievable by the PCR. However, if one uses a second set of primers that match the virus sequence, but which are different from those used in the first PCR reaction, i.e. hybridizing to viral sequences that lie within the outer primer pair, it is possible to amplify the target sequence further (*Figure 2*). The net effect of this second reaction is an overall increase in sensitivity and specificity of the PCR (*Protocol 6*), producing a 10 000-fold increase in amplification over that achieved by the outer primers alone (60).

Protocol 6. Nested PCR method[a]

Equipment and reagents

- PCR reagents: as for *Protocol 4*[b]
- 1.5% agarose[c] gel in TBE (see *Protocol 5*), pre-stained with 0.66 μg/ml ethidium bromide (**note: ethidium bromide is highly mutagenic, so always wear gloves when handling gels or solutions that contain ethidium bromide**)
- 1 × TBE electrophoresis buffer, containing 0.66 μg/ml ethidium bromide

- Size markers spanning expected size of second PCR product (e.g. plasmid DNA, such as pBR322 digested with *Hae*III, Boehringer cat. no. 821705)
- Ultraviolet light box
- Protective goggles or (preferably) full face mask

Method

1. For each reaction, prepare 20 μl reaction buffer containing:
   - 2 μl of PCR buffer (10 ×)
   - 17.7 μl of water
   - 0.1 μl of a 0.01 μg/ml Orange G dye solution in water
   - 0.2 μl of nucleoside triphosphate mixture
   - 0.1 μl of inner sense primer (1.5–6 pmol)
   - 0.1 μl of inner antisense primer
   - 0.4 units of *Taq* polymerase (0.05–0.2 μl)
   - 1 μl[d] of amplified DNA from *Protocol 4*

   Cover with a drop of mineral oil.

2. Transfer to a thermal cycler set with the times, temperatures, and numbers of cycles as in *Protocol 4*.

Protocol 6. *Continued*

3. After amplification, analyse entire sample by agarose gel electrophoresis, along with size markers. For speed and convenience:
    (a) Fill electrophoresis tank up to the top of the agarose gel, avoiding flooding the sample wells.
    (b) Add each sample, avoiding the paraffin layer (gel loading buffer not required).
    (c) Electrophorese samples at approximately 5 V/cm for 2–3 min.
    (d) Switch off power; add sufficient electrophoresis buffer to cover gel and flood wells.
    (e) Electrophorese at the same voltage for a further 5–10 min.
    (f) View gel on ultraviolet light box. Bands ranging in size from 100 to 500 bp will be resolved adequately by this procedure. As the sample is only run a short distance, it is possible to use several banks of sample combs with each agarose gel. Using the Pharmacia Horizontal Electrophoresis Tank (GNA 200), for example, it is possible to analyse approximately 250 samples (using eleven 22-well combs) on a single gel.

[a] Based on method described in reference 60.
[b] Note that this reaction should be set up in the general laboratory area using a separate set of reagents from those used for setting up the first PCR (see Sections 2.1.2 and 2.1.3).
[c] High concentrations of agarose impair the transparency of the gel. Low melting point agarose produces clearer gels, but is more expensive and is not necessary unless gels are to be photographed.
[d] Most laboratory workers experience the urge to add more than 1 μl to the second PCR. In fact, 1 μl is more than adequate: addition of larger amounts will lead to the appearance of multiple non-specific bands in the product, which can reduce the sensitivity of the PCR.

4.5.1 Evaluation of sensitivity of nested PCR

Before using nested primers for amplification of viral sequences in clinical specimens, it is recommended that a series of titrations be carried with known concentrations of target DNA to evaluate the performance of the assay (see Section 4.4). *Figure 3* shows the results of a titration of a recombinant HIV sequence, pBH10.R3, amplified by nested primers in the conserved *gag* region of the genome (60). While 65 fg of target DNA yielded a visible band after the first round of amplification (lane 3), as little as 6.5 ag (6.5×10^{-18} g) produced a positive signal after the second round (lane 7). The negative control that contained 1 μg of herring sperm DNA was completely negative after the second round of amplification (lane 9). The mass of one molecule of the target DNA used in this titration (pBH10.R3) was 13 ag (10 000 bp × 660 g/bp mol, divided by Avogadro's number), thus the amount detected at the final dilution may have been as little as one molecule.

4.5.2 Quantification of target DNA by nested PCR

To investigate the sensitivity of the PCR further, replicates containing different nominal amounts of target sequence were amplified by the nested PCR

Table 1. Frequency of positives with different amounts of target DNA

Input amount of pBH10.R3 [a] (ag) [e]	Observed frequency positives [b]	Average no. of input copies [c]	Estimated no. of copies per reaction [d]	Efficiency of amplification (%)
104	6/6	8	n/a [f]	n/a
52	11/12	4	2.49	62
26	6/12	2	0.69	35
13	6/12	1	0.69	69
6.5	7/19	0.5	0.46	92
3.25	4/18	0.25	0.25	100
1.63	2/18	0.13	0.12	92
0.81	0/18	0.06	0	n/a
0 (negative control)	0/40	0	0	n/a

[a] pBH10.R3 is a recombinant plasmid containing a nearly full-length HIV-1 genome. Purified plasmid was quantified by absorbance measurement at 260 nm, and serially diluted in TE buffer, supplemented with 200 μg/ml of sonicated herring sperm DNA/ml, to give the indicated amounts of target DNA in the 5 μl sample.
[b] Number of positive reactions over number of replicates tested obtained by amplification with nested primers in the *gag* region.
[c] Predicted number of molecules in sample from column 1.
[d] Calculated number of molecules in sample, using Poisson formula $-(\ln f_o)$.
[e] 1 ag $= 10^{-18}$ g.
[f] Not applicable.

protocol, and the products analysed by agarose gel electrophoresis (60; *Figure 3C*; *Table 1*). As can be seen, testing multiple replicates of 6.5 ag amounts of target DNA yielded some positive signals and some negatives (*Figure 3C*). The frequency of positives varied with the amount of target DNA amplified (*Table 1*).

In *Table 1*, the observed frequencies were converted into molecular concentrations of target DNA by the Poisson formula, $-(\ln f_o)$, where f_o is the frequency of negative reactions. The fourth column of *Table 1* gives the observed numbers of molecules at each dilution of DNA, and compares them (final column) with the calculated number (column 3). The similarity provides good evidence that the nested PCR can detect single molecules of target DNA, even when diluted in relatively large amounts of complex, non-target carrier DNA. This degree of sensitivity has been routinely achieved with several sets of HIV-specific primers, as well as those for HBV and parvovirus B19 (unpublished data).

The sensitivity of the nested PCR for single molecules of target DNA permits a straightforward method of quantification of viral sequences. In this method, test samples are titrated to an end-point; the final concentration producing a visible signal can be considered to contain at least one molecule of target. The accuracy of the titration can be increased to any degree of

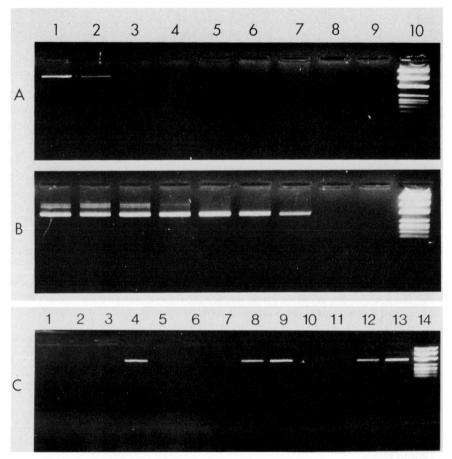

Figure 3. Titration and quantification of viral DNA sequences by nested PCR (reproduced from Ref. 60 with permission of the American Society for Microbiology). (A and B) Dilution series of recombinant HIV-1 DNA amplified by outer *gag* primers (A), followed by amplification of 1 μl of product with inner *gag* primers (B). (pBH10.R3, diluted in 200 μg/ml of herring sperm DNA; 1 μg/reaction). Lanes 1, 6.5 pg of DNA (5×10^5 copies); lanes 2, 650 fg (5×10^4 copies); lanes 3, 65 fg (5000 copies); lanes 4, 6.5 fg (500 copies); lanes 5, 650 ag (50 copies); lanes 6, 65 ag (5 copies); lanes 7, 6.5 ag (0.5 copies); lanes 8, 0.65 ag (0.05 copies); lanes 9, 1 μg of herring sperm DNA; lanes 10, molecular size markers (pTZ18R, digested with *Hae*II). (C) Limiting dilution: amplification of replicate samples each nominally containing 0.5 molecules of target HIV-1 sequence with nested *gag* primers (6.5 ag of pBH10.R3; lanes 2–12). Lane 1: negative control (1 μg of herring sperm DNA); lane 13: positive control (65 ag of pBH10.R3); lane 14: molecular size markers. See *Table 1* for frequencies of positives at other input HIV DNA concentrations.

precision by increasing the numbers of replicates at each dilution. The Poisson formula can then be applied to the resulting distribution of positive and negative results as described above to obtain a molecular concentration of DNA. A good compromise between accuracy of titration, and number of separate amplifications that need to be carried out, is to amplify a series of five-fold dilutions in triplicate. Another (preferred) approach is to titrate samples (very roughly) in 10-fold steps, and then to test multiple replicates of 2- to 5-fold dilutions around the cut-off point for greater accuracy. As will be discussed in Section 5, having some idea of the amount of viral RNA or DNA in a sample is often vital for interpretation in many diagnostic situations.

Levels of RNA in a sample can also be determined by titration of cDNA prepared from a suitable concentration of viral RNA in *Protocol 3*. However, as described above, not all of the RNA is reverse transcribed sufficiently far to allow amplification. The reader should consult reference 33 for more information on the efficiency of reverse transcription and amplification of primers with spacings that range from 250 to 800 base pairs. Quantification of HCV in plasma by this method is described in reference 61.

4.6 Advantages and disadvantages of different detection methods

Table 2 summarizes the principal advantages and disadvantages of detection methods for amplified DNA.

Table 2. Summary of PCR product detection methods

Method	Advantages	Disadvantages
Agarose gel electrophoresis, ethidium bromide staining	Quick, inexpensive	Extremely insensitive, non-specific, not generally suitable for virological detection.
Hybridization/ Southern blotting	Sensitive (can detect 10 copies of target DNA); positive identification of target DNA	Requires additional equipment, some protocols require expensive, hazardous, and short-lived radiolabel (^{32}P); requires optimization for maximum sensitivity; time-consuming.
Nested PCR	Highly sensitive, does not require optimization, high specificity, permits simple quantification by titration, requires no extra equipment, substantially reduced risk of contamination by product carry-over; generates large amounts of pure DNA that can be directly analysed (33, 60)	Amplification depends on correct matches of four, rather than two, primer pairs

4.7 Purification of PCR product

None of the simple DNA detection methods described above require any form of PCR product purification prior to analysis. However, one of the major applications of the PCR is the analysis of amplified DNA by restriction endonuclease site polymorphisms or nucleotide sequencing (see Section 5.1). The extent to which amplified DNA needs to be purified is dependent on what type of analysis is to be performed. Most restriction enzymes and DNA ligases do not work optimally, if at all, in PCR buffer, and it is recommended that some form of purification be carried out prior to enzyme digestion. Sequencing reactions are highly sensitive to impurities, residual primers, and nucleotide triphosphates present in the PCR mixture.

One of the simplest and most convenient methods of purification is ethanol precipitation. To the PCR product, add 400 µl of chloroform and remove the upper aqueous layer containing the amplified DNA. To this add two volumes of ice-cold 100% ethanol, mix, and spin at 14 000 g for 10 min to precipitate the DNA. Remove ethanol by aspiration and resuspend pellet containing the viral DNA in a small volume of water or TE buffer. DNA prepared in this manner should be cleavable by the majority of restriction enzymes.

For direct sequencing of double-stranded PCR product, higher purity is necessary. A convenient method is to extract the DNA with glass milk, such as 'Gene-Clean' (Bio 101), following the manufacturers' instructions (it is recommended that the mineral oil overlay is removed by the chloroform treatment described above before commencing the extraction). This method is unsuitable for extraction of single-stranded DNA, such as that generated by asymmetric PCR methods (63). Filtration of amplified DNA through 'Centricon' filters (Amicon) is effective for purification of both single- and double-stranded amplified DNA prior to sequencing.

PCR product may contain variable amounts of non-specifically amplified DNA that may interfere with restriction enzyme or sequence analysis. To remove this, electrophorese the PCR product on a pre-stained, low melting point agarose gel in a non-borate buffer (TAE buffer made from a 50 × stock solution of 2 M Tris–acetate (pH 8.0), 0.05 M EDTA (pH 8.0), diluted in distilled water is a suitable alternative for the agarose gel and running buffer). When the band corresponding to amplified viral DNA has migrated at least 5 cm, excise band from the gel with a razor blade in as small a piece of agarose as possible (**caution: unprotected areas of skin can be burnt by prolonged exposure to ultraviolet light. If possible, use full mask rather than goggles for this procedure**). DNA can now be extracted from the agarose using glass milk (see above).

5. Applications of PCR

The methods described in this chapter have the primary aim of allowing the sensitive and specific detection of viral sequences in clinical specimens.

However, in many cases, simple demonstration of the presence of viral DNA or RNA in a specimen is not sufficient. For example, the amount of virus in a specimen may be relevant when monitoring serial samples from a patient for evidence of virus reactivation during immunosuppression (64), HIV-related disease progression (60, 33), or response to antiviral treatment (65).

5.1 Analysis of viral sequence variation

It is often important clinically to differentiate virus types, such as distinguishing the carcinoma-associated HPV types 16 and 18 from the more common, assumed less sinister types. The use of type-specific primers has been discussed and examples given of their clinical application (Section 1.3.3).

Another method for typing viruses is to amplify samples with 'conserved' type-common primers that match all sequence variants of a particular virus, and then to analyse the amplified viral DNA between the primers for type-specific differences. Analysis of amplified viral DNA can be carried out by direct sequencing or analysis of restriction endonuclease site polymorphisms. This latter technique is particularly suitable for diagnostic purposes, as it is quick to carry out and needs little extra apparatus (66–68). Restriction endonucleases have also been used for analysis of sequence diversity and 'molecular' epidemiological studies of several human viruses (69–74), and as a method for positive identification of amplified DNA as being of viral origin (74–77). These papers should be referred to for further practical information.

5.2 Examples of current diagnostic uses of PCR

One of the most important current applications of PCR is in the diagnosis of infection in the neonate, particularly of viral infections that may require urgent clinical intervention in the neonatal period e.g. herpes simplex virus (78) and varicella-zoster virus. The PCR may provide the only evidence of vertical transmission of viruses that cannot be reliably isolated (e.g. HIV (79) and rubella (80)), in the 12–18 month period in which the use of conventional serological assays is precluded by the presence of passively acquired maternal antibody. In the same way as the PCR has been used for the antenatal diagnosis of inherited disease, fetal sampling may be used to diagnose intra-uterine infection. This would be especially important for rubella and other viruses causing congenital malformations.

Another example where virus isolation may be unreliable and/or too slow, and serological methods of diagnosis of no use, is in the diagnosis and treatment of viral encephalitis or meningitis. Reports of the detection of HSV (62, 50) and enteroviruses (81) by PCR at the onset of disease in the cerebrospinal fluid of patients with encephalitis or meningitis will allow earlier and more definitive diagnoses to be made.

The examples given on virus detection, quantification, and sequence variation illustrate how the PCR may provide diagnostic information of immediate practical importance. Whereas one has to caution against the over-use of PCR in situations where existing methods are perfectly adequate, the sheer pace of developments in this field indicates that the PCR will probably become one of the mainstays of viral diagnosis in the future.

Acknowledgements

The author is indebted to Dr L. Q. Zhang, Dr A. J. Leigh Brown, A. Cleland, and S. Ashelford at the IACPB, Division of Biology, and Dr S. W. Chan and F. McOmish at the Department of Medical Microbiology, University of Edinburgh, for providing valuable practical information in the protocols, and critical discussion of the chapter as it was written. Thanks are also due to Dr M. O. Ogilvie for information and discussion of the clinical application of PCR, both current and future.

Since the submission of this manuscript, PCR kits for various applications have become commercially available. Those are not discussed in detail here, but should be used and judged according to principles and problems as outlined in this chapter.

References

1. Saiki, R. K., Scharf, S. J., Faloona, F. A., Mullis, K. B., Horn, G. T., Erlich, H. A., and Arnheim, N. (1985). *Science*, **230**, 1350.
2. Mullis, K., Faloona, F., Scharf, S., Saiki, R., Horn, G., and Erlich, H. (1986). *Cold Spring Harbor Symp. Quant. Biol.*, **51**, 263.
3. Scharf, S. J., Horn, G. T., and Erlich, H. A. (1986). *Science*, **233**, 1076.
4. Mullis, K. B. and Faloona, F. A. (1987). In *Methods in Enzymology* (ed. R. Wu) Vol. 155, pp. 335–50. Academic Press, London.
5. Kwok, S. Y., Mack, D. H., Mullis, K. B., Poiesz, B. J., Ehrlich, G. D., Blair, D., *et al.* (1987). *J. Virol.*, **61**, 1690.
6. Ou, C.-Y., Kwok, S., Mitchell, S. W., Mack, D. H., Sninsky, J. J., Krebs, J. W., *et al.* (1988). *Science*, **239**, 295.
7. Chien, A., Edgar, D. B., and Trela, J. M. (1976). *J. Bacteriol.*, **127**, 1550.
8. Saiki, R. K., Gelfand, D. H., Stoffel, S., Scharf, S. J., Higuchi, R. G., Horn, G. T., *et al.* (1988). *Science*, **239**, 487.
9. Elie, C., Salhi, S., Rossignol, J. M., Forterre, P., and de Recondo, A. M. (1988). *Biochim. Biophys. Acta*, **951**, 261.
10. Fiala, G. and Stetter, K. O. (1986). *Arch. Microbiol.*, **145**, 56.
11. Eckert, K. A. and Kunkle, T. A. (1990). *Nucleic Acids Res.*, **18**, 3739.
12. Williams, P., Simmonds, P., Yap, P. L., Balfe, P., Bishop, J., Brettle, R., *et al.* (1990). *AIDS*, **4**, 393.
13. Leigh Brown, A. J. and Monaghan, P. (1988). *AIDS Res. Hum. Retrovir.*, **4**, 399.
14. McNicol, P. J. and Dodd, J. G. (1990). *J. Clin. Microbiol.*, **28**, 409.
15. Resnick, R. M., Cornelissen, M. T., Wright, D. K., Eichinger, G. H., Fox, H. S., ter Schegget, J., and Manos, M. M. (1990). *J. Natl. Cancer Inst.*, **82**, 1477–84.

16. Kimura, H., Shibata, M., Kuzushima, K., Nishikawa, K., Nishiyama, Y., and Morishima, T. (1990). *Med. Microbiol. Immunol. (Berlin)*, **179**, 177.
17. Norder, H., Hammas, B., and Magnius, L. O. (1990). *J. Med. Virol.*, **31**, 215.
18. Gouvea, V., Glass, R. I., Woods, P., Taniguchi, K., Clark, H. F., Forrester, B., and Fang, Z. Y. (1990). *J. Clin. Microbiol.*, **28**, 276.
19. Kwok, S. and Higuchi, R. (1989). *Nature*, **339**, 237.
20. Sarkar, G. and Sommer, S. S. (1990). *Nature*, **343**, 27.
21. Garson, J. A., Tuke, P. W., Makris, M., Briggs, M., Machin, S. J., Preston, F. E., and Tedder, R. S. (1990). *Lancet*, **336**, 1022.
22. Jansen, R. W., Siegl, G., and Lemon, S. M. (1990). *Proc. Natl. Acad. Sci. USA*, **87**, 2867.
23. Brown, V. K. and Robertson, B. H. (1990). *Biotechniques*, **8**, 262.
24. Zeldis, J. B., Lee, J. H., Mamish, D., Finegold, D. J., Sircar, R., Ling, Q., et al. (1989). *J. Clin. Invest.*, **84**, 1503.
25. Harding, J. D., Gebeyehu, G., Bebee, R., Simms, D., and Klevan, L. (1989). *Nucleic Acids Res.*, **17**, 6947.
26. Yamada, O., Matsumoto, T., Nakashima, M., Hagari, S., Kamahora, T., Ueyama, H., et al. (1990). *J. Virol. Methods*, **27**, 203.
27. Albert, J. and Fenyö, E. M. (1990). *J. Clin. Microbiol.*, **28**, 1560.
28. Cheyrou, A., Guyomarc'h, C., and Blouin, P. (1991). *Nucleic Acids Res.*, **19**, 4006.
29. Kim, H. S. and Smithies, O. (1988). *Nucleic Acids Res.*, **16**, 8887.
30. Kaneko, S., Feinstone, S. M., and Miller, R. H. (1989). *J. Clin. Microbiol.*, **27**, 1930.
31. Sambrook, J., Fritsch, E. F., and Maniatis, T. (1989). *Molecular cloning. A laboratory manual*, 2nd edn. Cold Spring Harbor Laboratory Press, Cold Spring Harbor, NY.
32. Ausubel, F. M., Brent, R., Kingston, R. E., Moore, D. D., Seidman, J. G., Smith, J. A., and Struhl, K. (1987). *Current protocols in molecular biology*. Wiley Interscience, New York.
33. Zhang, L. Q., Simmonds, P., Ludlam, C. A., and Leigh Brown, A. J. (1991). *AIDS*, **5**, 675.
34. Chomczynski, P. and Sacchi, N. (1987). *Anal. Biochem.*, **162**, 156.
35. Dangler, C. A., de Mattos, C. A., de Mattos, C. C., and Osburn, B. I. (1990). *J. Virol. Methods*, **28**, 281.
36. Davis, V. S. and Boyle, J. A. (1990). *Anal. Biochem.*, **189**, 30.
37. Longo, M. C., Berninger, M. S., and Hartley, J. L. (1990). *Gene*, **93**, 125.
38. Cimino, G. D., Metchette, K. C., Tessman, J. W., Hearst, J. E., and Isaacs, S. T. (1991). *Nucleic Acids Res.*, **19**, 99.
39. Kumar, R., Goedert, J. J., and Hughes, S. H. (1989). *AIDS Res. Hum. Retrovir.*, **5**, 345.
40. Coutlee, F., Bobo, L., Mayur, K., Yolken, R. H., and Viscidi, R. P. (1989). *Anal. Biochem.*, **181**, 96.
41. Coutlee, F., Yang, B. Z., Bobo, L., Mayur, K., Yolken, R., and Viscidi, R. (1990). *AIDS Res. Hum. Retrovir.*, **6**, 775.
42. Inouye, S. and Hondo, R. (1990). *J. Clin. Microbiol.*, **28**, 1469.
43. Keller, G. H., Huang, D. P., Shih, J. W., and Manak, M. M. (1990). *J. Clin. Microbiol.*, **28**, 1411.

44. Loche, M. and Mach, B. (1988). *Lancet*, **ii**, 418.
45. Bolton, E. T. and McCarthy, B. J. (1962). *Proc. Natl. Acad. Sci. USA*, **48**, 1390.
46. Bonner, T. I., Brenner, D. J., Neufeld, B. R., and Britten, R. J. (1973). *J. Mol. Biol.*, **81**, 123.
47. Arthur, R. R., Dagostin, S., and Shah, K. V. (1989). *J. Clin. Microbiol.*, **27**, 1174.
48. Kaneko, S., Miller, R. H., Feinstone, S. M., Unoura, M., Kobayashi, K., Hattori, N., and Purcell, R. H. (1989). *Proc. Natl. Acad. Sci. USA*, **86**, 312.
49. Olive, D. M., Simsek, M., and al Mufti, S. (1989). *J. Clin. Microbiol.*, **27**, 1238.
50. Puchhammer-Stockl, E., Popow-Kraupp, T., Heinz, F. X., Mandl, C. W., and Kunz, C. (1990). *J. Med. Virol.*, **32**, 77.
51. Arrigo, S. J., Weitsman, S., Zack, J. A., and Chen, I. S. (1990). *J. Virol.*, **64**, 4585.
52. Katz, J. P., Bodin, E. T., and Coen, D. M. (1990). *J. Virol.*, **64**, 4288.
53. Zack, J. A., Arrigo, S. J., Weitsman, S. R., Go, A. S., Haislip, A. and Chen, I. S. (1990). *Cell*, **61**, 213.
54. Oka, S., Urayama, K., Hirabayashi, Y., Ohnishi, K., Goto, H., Mitamura, K., *et al.* (1990). *Biochem. Biophys. Res. Commun.*, **167**, 1.
55. Pang, S., Koyanagi, Y., Miles, S., Wiley, C., Vinters, H. V., and Chen, I. S. (1990). *Nature*, **343**, 85.
56. Kellogg, D. E., Sninsky, J. J., and Kwok, S. (1990). *Anal. Biochem.*, **189**, 202.
57. Okamoto, H., Yotsumoto, S., Tsuda, F., Machida, A., and Mayumi, M. (1989). *Jpn. J. Exp. Med.*, **59**, 259.
58. Wang, A. M., Doyle, M. V., and Mark, D. F. (1989). *Proc. Natl. Acad. Sci. USA*, **86**, 9717.
59. Gilliland, G., Perrin, S., Blanchard, K., and Bunn, H. F. (1990). *Proc. Natl. Acad. Sci. USA*, **87**, 2725.
60. Simmonds, P., Balfe, P., Peutherer, J. F., Ludlam, C. A., Bishop, J. O., and Brown, A. J. (1990). *J. Virol.*, **64**, 864.
61. Simmonds, P., Zhang, L. Q., Watson, H. G., Rebus, S., Ferguson, E. D., Balfe, P., *et al.* (1990). *Lancet*, **336**, 1469.
62. Aurelius, E., Johansson, B., Skoldenberg, B., Staland, A., and Forsgren, M. (1991). *Lancet*, **337**, 189.
63. Gyllensten, U. B. and Erlich, H. A. (1988). *Proc. Natl. Acad. Sci. USA*, **85**, 7652.
64. Gerna, G., Parea, M., Percivalle, E., Zipeto, D., Silini, E., Barbarini, G., and Milanesi, G. (1990). *AIDS*, **4**, 1027.
65. Brillanti, S., Garson, J. A., Tuke, P. W., Ring, C., Briggs, M., Masci, C., *et al.* (1991). *J. Med. Virol.*, **34**, 136–41.
66. Shih, J. W. K., Ling, C. C., Alter, H. J., Lee, L. M., and Gu, J. R. (1991). *J. Clin. Microbiol.*, **29**, 1640.
67. Sample, J., Young, L., Martin, B., Chatman, T., Kieff, E., and Rickinson, A. (1990). *J. Virol.*, **64**, 4084.
68. Lunkenheimer, K., Hufert, F. T., and Schmitz, H. (1990). *J. Clin. Microbiol.*, **28**, 2689.
69. Liang, T. J., Blum, H. E., and Wands, J. R. (1990). *Hepatology*, **12**, 204.
70. Taylor, M. J., Godfrey, E., Baczko, K., ter Meulen, V., Wild, T. F., and Rima, B. K. (1991). *J. Gen. Virol.*, **72**, 83.
71. Xia, Y. P., Chang, M. F., Wei, D., Govindarajan, S., and Lai, M. M. (1990). *Virology*, **178**, 331.

72. Yanagihara, R., Nerurkar, V. R., Garruto, R. M., Miller, M. A., Leon-Monzon, M. E., Jenkins, C. L., *et al.* (1991). *Proc. Natl. Acad. Sci. USA*, **88**, 1446.
73. Cane, P. A. and Pringle, C. R. (1991). *J. Gen. Virol.*, **72**, 349.
74. Smith, J. S., Fishbein, D. B., Rupprecht, C. E., and Clark, K. (1991). *N. Engl. J. Med.*, **324**, 205.
75. Godec, M. S., Asher, D. M., Swoveland, P. T., Eldadah, Z. A., Feinstone, S. M., Goldfarb, L. G., *et al.* (1990). *J. Med. Virol.*, **30**, 237.
76. Maes, R. K., Beisel, C. E., Spatz, S. J., and Thacker, B. J. (1990). *Vet. Microbiol.*, **24**, 281.
77. Carman, W. F., Williamson, C., Cunliffe, B. A., and Kidd, A. H. (1989). *J. Virol. Methods*, **25**, 21.
78. Kimura, H., Fatamura, M., Kito, H., Ando, T., Goto, M., Kuzushima, K., *et al.* (1991). *J. Infect. Dis.*, **164**, 289.
79. Rogers, M. F., Ou, C. Y., Rayfield, M., Thomas, P. A., Schoenbaum, E. E., Abrams, E., *et al.* (1989). *N. Engl. J. Med.*, **320**, 1649.
80. Ho-Terry, L., Terry, G. M., and Londesborough, P. (1990). *J. Gen. Virol.*, **71**, 1607.
81. Rotbart, H. A. (1990). *J. Pediatr.*, **117**, 85.

6

Design and testing of antiviral compounds

DEREK KINCHINGTON, HILLAR KANGRO, and
DONALD J. JEFFRIES

1. Introduction

The search for antiviral drugs began in earnest in the 1950s but this was directed mainly by chance, with little or no scientific basis. Early successes included the use of methisazone (Marboran) for the prophylaxis of smallpox (1) and the use of idoxuridine (IUDR) for the treatment of herpes keratitis. It was soon realized that viral DNA or RNA replication involved virus-specified enzymes which provided potential targets for intervention, and the main emphasis in drug development became centred on nucleoside analogues. Several active drugs were identified, mainly against herpesviruses, but because of cellular toxicity their clinical usefulness was limited. A major breakthrough came in the late 1970s with the discovery of acyclovir (ACV; see reference 2), the most effective and least toxic antiviral drug developed so far. More recently a drug related to acyclovir, ganciclovir, has emerged which is effective against cytomegalovirus (CMV; see reference 3). The nucleoside analogue azidothymidine (AZT) has been developed for the treatment of human immunodeficiency virus (HIV) infections (4). The antiviral drugs in current use are summarized in *Table 1*. With the recent technological advances in molecular biology and ultrastructural analysis to aid in drug development, we can now be optimistic about the future role of chemotherapy in the control and treatment of virus disease. It may be possible to target biochemical pathways precisely in order to inhibit a virus or to restore the equilibrium of the cell disturbed by viral replication. The aim of this chapter is to describe in detail some of the laboratory methods currently used for assessing the activity and toxicity of potential antiviral compounds.

1.1 Targets for antiviral research

The relatively simple structure of viruses has not meant that they are easy targets for chemotherapy. In fact, the reverse is true: as the replication cycle of a virus is intimately associated with the host cell's biochemical pathways,

Table 1. Summary of currently used antiviral compounds

Compound	Mainly used against	IC_{50} (μM)[a]	Selectivity index[a]
Acyclovir	Herpes simplex virus,	0.1–1	>1000
	varicella-zoster virus	2–10	>1000
Ganciclovir	Cytomegalovirus,	2–10	100–1000
	herpes simplex virus	0.2–2	100–1000
Vidarabine	Herpes simplex virus,	10–40	50–100
	varicella-zoster virus	10–50	50–100
Idoxuridine	Herpes simplex virus (ocular)	0.3–5	<10
Trifluorothymidine	Herpes simplex virus (ocular)	0.3–5	<10
Azidothymidine	Human immunodeficiency virus	0.03–0.5	>1000
Dideoxycytidine	Human immunodeficiency virus	0.5–1.5	100–1000
Dideoxyinosine	Human immunodeficiency virus	2–10	$\geq$100
Phosphonoformate	Herpesviruses	20–200	1000
Amantadine	Influenza A virus	0.5–5	10–100
Rimantadine	Influenza A virus	0.05–1	50–100
Ribavirin	Respiratory syncytial viral	4–40	$\geq$10 000

[a] Can vary significantly depending on virus strain and cell type for culture. Figures shown are commonly published ranges with commonly used cell cultures, for comparative purposes. For IC_{50} determination see *Protocol 6* and *Figure 5*.

good selectivity has been difficult to achieve. Some viruses persist as a latent infection, in which case antiviral drugs are less likely to be effective. However, increased understanding of the molecular events of virus infections has meant that the search for antiviral drugs, against specific targets, can be conducted on a more rational basis. This approach has led to the discovery of a number of compounds active against herpesvirus enzymes involved in DNA replication and to the synthesis of proteinase inhibitors for HIV (5). With more detailed information of how drugs act at the molecular level, it may be possible to improve efficacy further and to combat the increasing problems of drug resistance in patients on long-term treatment.

The DNA polymerase of herpes simplex virus (HSV) provides a major target for antiviral drugs. It is essential for viral replication and can be inhibited by many compounds, including the nucleoside analogues ara-A and ACV. These compounds, which require conversion to the active triphosphates by phosphokinases, can act as chain terminators blocking extension of the replicating DNA molecule. In addition, DNA primers with ACV incorporated bind irreversibly to the polymerase, thus inactivating the enzyme. In comparison, Foscarnet (phosphonoformate; Astra Pharmaceuticals) is a pyrophosphate analogue and binds directly to the pyrophosphate binding site on the polymerase. Thus, it does not have to be activated or altered metabolically and provides an alternative means of inhibiting DNA replication. The direct action of polymerase binding by Foscarnet, avoiding the phosphokinase activity required to activate nucleoside analogues, has had clinical benefit since Foscarnet has been used successfully to treat ACV-resistant mutants of HSV. The HSV polymerase has been cloned and expressed in yeast cells which should allow molecular studies of drug activity and mechanisms of resistance. These studies on HSV mutants resistant to ACV due to changes in the polymerase gene have shown that this appears to be related to mutations in a small region of the carboxy-terminus of the enzyme; a highly conserved region showing homology with polymerases of other DNA viruses and human α-polymerase. The reverse transcriptase of HIV has been successfully cloned and expressed to enable studies on the activity of AZT and other drugs. It has been shown that AZT and Foscarnet bind directly to reverse transcriptase at sites which are in close proximity.

Although the main emphasis in drug development has been to find inhibitors targeted at specific viral enzymes involved in nucleic acid replication, such as reverse transcriptase, DNA polymerase, or thymidine kinase, all stages of the virus replication cycle are amenable to intervention. Thus, *in vitro* studies have shown that short peptides and soluble $CD4^+$ can be used to block adsorption of HIV. The drugs amantadine and rimantadine interfere with the penetration and uncoating of influenza A virus, possibly by raising the pH inside cytoplasmic vacuoles and thereby preventing the structural alterations of the viral haemagglutinin required for fusion and uncoating. In addition, amantadine blocks the later stages of virus assembly and release. The drug is thought to interfere with interactions between the viral M2 protein (membrane protein) and the viral haemagglutinin, thereby disrupting the envelopment of the nucleocapsid and hence reducing infectivity. Mutants resistant to amantadine, through alterations in the M2 protein, can be generated in the laboratory (6). Interferon and thiosemicarbazones interfere with the translation of viral proteins by affecting polysomal complexes and reducing mRNA stability. In recent years it has been shown that even mature virions can provide a target for antiviral drugs (see below).

1.2 Molecular graphics

For a number of years it has been possible to determine the structure of molecules which form regular crystalline arrays, firstly by electron microscopy but more recently by analysis of their diffraction patterns when placed in a beam of radiation. The most recent application of diffraction has employed X-rays with a wavelength of about 0.1 nm, and this has made it possible to deduce the arrangement of individual atoms in molecules from which the crystal is built. The analysis of diffraction patterns gives the three-dimensional arrangement of atoms in a representative molecule. Two associated developments have contributed to the technology: the automated data collection on powerful computers together with improvements in growing crystals. With high-quality crystals a resolution of 0.3 nm is achievable, revealing the position of all the non-hydrogen atoms in the protein. This technique has been

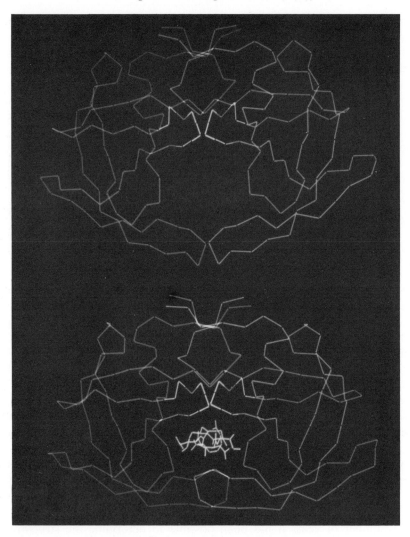

Figure 1. Diagram of three-dimensional structure of HIV-1 proteinase showing an inhibitor in the active site. (Courtesy Dr T. Krohn, Roche Products UK Ltd).

used successfully in the development of a novel proteinase inhibitor of HIV (*Figure 1*). Similarly, determination of the three-dimensional structure of rhinoviruses (7) has resulted in a series of compounds (disoxanil; also known as the 'WIN' series) which are targeted against mature extracellular virions. These drugs fit into a hydrophobic cleft structure formed on the surface of the virions by the folding of the VP1 structural polypeptide. Following entry of the virus into cells, this cleft structure normally collapses during uncoating but the effect of the 'WIN' drug is to immobilize the cleft, thereby preventing uncoating and release of the viral RNA (8).

1.3 Drug assessment

Two different approaches are available for investigating compounds that may be active against any particular virus. The first involves random screening of compounds, such as those isolated from plant extracts or from collections of chemically synthesized compounds, which may have been produced for other purposes. Those compounds which show activity may then be used to synthesize new analogues in an attempt to improve their antiviral activity. The second approach is to synthesize compounds which are designed to act on a specific viral target. The subsequent discovery of an active drug may involve a detailed analysis of structure–activity relationships of a series of derivatives together with an assessment of their toxicity in the target cells. The relationship between the antiviral activity and toxicity of a compound is given as its selectivity index (SI) (see *Table 1*).

$$SI = \frac{\text{drug concentration required to inhibit cell proliferation (or DNA synthesis)}}{\text{drug concentration required to inhibit virus replication}}$$

Usually a compound should have an SI of > 100 *in vitro* before it would be considered for further development.

2. Assays for virus infectivity

Before antiviral testing can be carried out, either to screen drugs for antiviral activity or to test clinical isolates for resistance to drugs, it is essential to obtain a seed stock of the virus with known infectivity. Virus infectivity is usually determined either as 50% tissue culture infective dose $(TCID)_{50}$ or as plaque forming units (p.f.u.). Both measure the amount of infectious units in a virus preparation. Examples of both assay methods are described below. (*Protocols 1* and *2*)

2.1 Determination of the TCID$_{50}$ of HIV1 in C8166 T-lymphoblastoid cells

The TCID$_{50}$ is determined in replicate cultures of serial dilutions of the stock virus preparations (clarified culture supernatant). The titre of the virus stock is expressed as the TCID$_{50}$ which can be calculated more accurately than a negative end-point. This method is outlined in *Protocol 1*.

Protocol 1.

1. Mark up a 96-well, flat-bottom tissue culture plate so that the central 60 wells (10 horizontal and six vertical) are used. To each well add 2×10^4

Protocol 1. *Continued*

C8166 cells in 100 µl of culture medium (RPMI 1640 plus 10% bovine calf serum).

2. Prepare a tenfold dilution series from 10^{-1} to 10^{-9} of the original high titre virus stock in 1 ml volumes of culture medium in 4 ml plastic tubes. Add 100 µl of the high titre stock to the first column of wells and 100 µl of increasing virus dilutions to subsequent columns. Each well should contain 200 µl.

3. Add sterile (PBS) to the empty wells around the perimeter of the plate to reduce 'edge effects' due to evaporation and incubate at 37°C in 5% CO_2–air.

4. Inspect the plate daily for cytopathic effects (CPEs). The CPE caused by HIV-1 in C8166 cells is observed as formation of syncytia (multinucleated giant cells). Syncytia may form in the first row within a few hours if the titre of virus is high.

5. Remove 100 µl from each well after 3–4 days and re-feed with 100 µl of fresh culture medium if necessary (the normally pink medium will turn yellow as it becomes acid).

6. After 3–4 days, syncytia will be present in other wells. When no further CPE can be seen to develop (usually day 4 or 5) the number of replicate wells showing CPE is recorded for each virus dilution (*Table 2*).

7. The $TCID_{50}$, i.e. the concentration when 50% of cultures becomes infected, is calculated using the method of Reed and Muench (see reference 9). In this procedure the numbers of infected and uninfected cultures (wells) at each dilution are compared and the dilution giving 50% infected wells is estimated.

In the example shown in *Table 2*, none of the dilutions gives a 50% end-point; in this case the end-point lies between dilutions 10^{-7} and 10^{-8}. A simple interpolation of the proportionate distance is used to determine the 50% end-point.

Proportionate distance =

$$\frac{(\% \text{ infected wells at next dilution above } 50\%) - (50\%)}{(\% \text{ infected wells at next dilution above } 50\%) - (\% \text{ infected wells at next dilution below } 50\%)} \times n$$

(where n = the log of dilution step, which in this case is log 1/10 = −1)

$$= \frac{66.7 - 50}{66.7 - 22.2} = 0.38n = -0.38$$

Thus the log $TCID_{50}$ is −7 + (−0.38) = −7.38. The $TCID_{50}$ is $10^{-7.38}$, and the virus stock is said to contain $10^{7.38}$ $TCID_{50}$ of virus.

The assays can also be carried out in 24-well cluster plates with 2 ml

Table 2. Results obtained in a titration of a suspension of HIV in cell culture

Virus dilution	Observed values		Accumulated values		
	Wells +	Wells −	Wells +	Wells −	% Infected
10^{-5}	6	0	17	0	100
10^{-6}	5	1	11	1	91.6
10^{-7}	4	2	6	3	66.6
10^{-8}	2	4	2	7	22.2
10^{-9}	0	6	0	13	0

(containing 2×10^5 cells) per well. The advantage of the larger volumes is that it reduces the likelihood of edge effects.

2.2 Plaque method for determining virus infectivity

Plaques are discrete regions of virus growth within monolayer cultures and reflect the cytopathic behaviour of a particular virus. They may appear as foci of transformed cells, as multinucleated cells, areas of dead cells, or gaps in the monolayer from which dead cells have detached. By counting the number of plaques, an estimate can be obtained of the number of infectious units present in a virus preparation (see *Protocol 2*). Seed stocks of virus can be prepared from standard laboratory strains or clinical isolates by harvesting culture supernatants or sonication of infected cells. The virus preparation is clarified by centrifugation and stored at $-70\,^{\circ}$C in aliquots. It is important to remember that if frozen virus stocks are to be used in the drug assay, the stock should be titrated after freezing/thawing it once. Titration of a stock of herpes simplex virus (HSV) is conveniently done in a 24-well cluster plate.

Protocol 2.

1. Feed 24-well plates with 2×10^5 Vero cells/ml and incubate at $37\,^{\circ}$C in 5% CO_2 in air until confluent.

2. Prepare serial 10-fold dilutions of the stock of HSV in culture medium (medium 199 with Earle's salt, 1% fetal calf serum, 0.22% bicarbonate, 2mM glutamine, 100 u/ml penicillin, 100 µg/ml streptomycin) and inoculate 0.5 ml of each dilution into each of two replicate wells per dilution. Incubate for 1 h at $37\,^{\circ}$C in 5% CO_2 in air to allow adsorption of the virus.

3. Remove the inoculum and re-feed with 'overlay medium'. The overlay medium consists of maintenance medium with 1% carboxymethyl cellulose (CMC) or 0.5% agarose (preferably low melting point). High titre neutralizing serum can be added in place of CMC or agarose. The overlay medium or neutralizing serum is added to prevent secondary plaque formation from progeny virus released into the medium during

---

Protocol 2. *Continued*

incubation. This procedure may not be necessary for viruses with a long replication cycle (such as CMV or varicella-zoster virus) but the overlay medium is still usually added as a precaution and because plaque formation is sometimes improved.

4. Remove the 'overlay medium' by suction after 48–72 h incubation and fix the cell sheets with 10% formalin in PBS for 30 min at ambient temperature.

5. Rinse the wells with water and stain the cell sheets with 0.5% crystal violet in methanol:water (20:80, v/v) for 20 minutes. Rinse the cell sheets with plenty of tap water and leave the plates to dry on the bench.

6. Count the number of plaques while viewing with a binocular microscope or a magnifying box. Choose the wells which contain a high enough dilution of the virus stock to give discrete plaques (usually <100 per well). This gives a direct measure of the virus titre as p.f.u. per ml. For drug assays, a dilution of the seed stock is usually chosen to give 20–40 plaques per well.

3. Toxicity testing in cell culture

The preliminary evaluation of new drugs often starts with screening for toxicity in the culture system to be used. This ensures that the drugs will eventually be tested in the appropriate concentration range when tested against the virus. A crude measure of toxicity can be obtained simply by including a series of dilutions of the drug in maintenance medium added to cell cultures in cluster plates and observing the cells for evidence of toxicity. Staining of the cells with a vital stain after exposure to the drug (*Protocol 3*) can be used and is most suitable for assessing toxicity in cultures of non-adherent cells. However, repeated passage of cells in the presence of the compound, accompanied by total and viable cell counts (*Protocol 4*), provides a more discriminating method of detecting cytotoxicity. Many compounds can be excluded from further studies at this stage. Compounds which are not soluble in water are usually dissolved in dimethylsulphoxide (DMSO), and the final concentration of DMSO in the culture medium must be no more than 1%. The incorporation of radioactive precursors into nucleic acids or proteins (*Protocol 5*) is used to monitor low levels of toxicity.

Protocol 3. Vital staining with trypan blue

1. Resuspend cells in the appropriate volume of culture medium and pipette aliquots of 2×10^4 cells in 200 μl into a 96-well plate, or 2×10^5 cells into a 24-well plate.

2. Add compounds at the appropriate dilutions and incubate cells at 37 °C

in 5% CO_2 in air for 3–5 days. Compounds should be tested in replicate wells at each concentration.

3. Prepare a 10 ml stock solution of trypan blue (10 mg/ml) in PBS.

4. Resuspend cells in PBS to give 10^4–10^5 cells/ml, mix for example 0.25 ml with an equal volume of trypan blue and leave for 1 min. Count the number of live (unstained) and dead (blue) cells in the sample using a haemocytometer and calculate the percentage viability of cells at each dilution of the compound.

Protocol 4. Formazan method

This method is based on the fact that the yellow tetrazolium salt MTT [3-(4,5-dimethylthiazol-2-yl)-2,5-diphenyltetrazolium bromide] is converted to dark blue formazan by living cells but not by dead cells or culture medium. Assays are carried out in 96-well microplates.

1. Resuspend cells in the appropriate volume of culture medium and pipette aliquots of 2×10^4 cells in 200 µl into a 96-well plate.

2. Add compounds at the appropriate dilutions and incubate cells at 37 °C in 5% CO_2 in air for 3–5 days. Compounds should be tested in replicate wells at each concentration.

3. Add 10 µl of 5 mg/ml MTT to cells in 100 µl of culture fluid and incubate the plates in 5% CO_2 in air for a further 4 h.

4. Remove supernatants gently by pipetting, or after centrifugation at 800 g for 5 min (for non-adherent cells). This avoids occasional precipitation of serum proteins which may occur when the acid–alcohol mixture is added.

5. Add 150 µl of acid–isopropanol (0.04 M HCl in isopropanol) to all wells and mix thoroughly to dissolve the dark blue crystals of formazan which are formed.

6. Read the plates on a plate reader at 540 nm and with a reference wavelength of 690 nm. Subtract the absorbance measured at 690 nm from the absorbance at 540 nm, to eliminate the effects of non-specific absorbance. The 50% cytotoxic dose (CD_{50}) is given as the concentration of compound that reduces the absorbance (at 540 nm) of the uninfected cell samples by 50% (see reference 10).

A sensitive method to measure toxic effects of drugs is to monitor cellular metabolism by incorporation of [^{3}H]thymidine or ^{14}C-labelled protein hydrolysate (*Protocol 5*). ^{14}C-labelling of proteins is used in preference to [^{3}H]thymidine incorporation when competition between labelled and un-labelled nucleosides in cellular uptake has to be avoided. These methods are used mainly to monitor sub-lethal toxicity after initial screening or when comparing different metabolites in a series of related compounds. The assays can be carried out using 2×10^5 cells in 24-well plates or 6 ml culture tubes, or using 2×10^4 cells in 96-well plates.

Protocol 5. Incorporation of radiolabelled precursors

1. Incubate aliquots of uninfected cells in the presence of the compounds being tested at the appropriate concentrations for 72 h in 5% CO_2 in air. Include control wells without added compound.

2. Centrifuge the tubes or plates (1000 r.p.m.), if non-adherent cells are used, and remove the medium from each sample. Rinse cells twice with PBS and resuspend each cell sample in 200 μl of growth medium containing the radioisotope ([^{3}H]thymidine 1 μCi/ml; [^{14}C] labelled protein hydrolysate 0.25 μCi/ml). Incubate for 12–18 h at 37 °C in 5% CO_2 in air. At higher concentrations of the isotopes, cells may be harvested after 4–5 hours.

3. Harvest the cells on Whatman no. 3 paper using a cell harvester (Skatron). Rinse adherent cells with PBS and lyse with distilled water or detergent before spotting on to filter membranes.

4. Measure incorporated [^{3}H]thymidine or ^{14}C-labelled amino acids in a β-scintillation counter. Express the uptake of radioisotope in the treated cells as % incorporation of the untreated cells.

---

4. Measuring compound efficacy in cell culture

The activity of compounds on viruses is generally assessed by dose–response experiments. A standard virus preparation is incubated with indicator cells in the presence of increasing concentrations of compound to determine the concentration that will inhibit virus replication. The assays can be made quantitative by a number of methods, e.g. plaque counting, dye uptake, or virus antigen detection. The activity of the drug or the sensitivity of the virus isolate to a given drug is usually expressed as the concentration of drug required to inhibit virus replication by 50% (IC_{50}: 50% inhibitory concentration). *Protocols 6–9* give examples of the commonly used types of assays.

4.1 Plaque reduction assay

Protocol 6. Plaque reduction assay of inhibitory activity against herpes simplex virus

This is based on the plaque assay described in *Protocol 2*. An example of a plaque reduction assay for activity of ACV against HSV is shown in *Figure 2*.

1. Prepare cultures of confluent Vero cells in 24-well plates.

---

2. Dilute the virus seed stock to inoculate with 20–50 plaques per well, and incubate for 1 h to allow virus adsorption.

3. Prepare an appropriate dilution series of the antiviral compound in overlay medium (1% CMC or 0.5% agarose in Parker's 199 maintenance medium). Compounds with unknown activity should be screened initially over a wide range of concentrations e.g. 2, 20, or 200 μM.

4. Remove the virus and re-feed the cell sheets with overlay medium containing the antiviral compound under test (1 ml/well). Prepare replicate wells for each dilution of compound and include virus controls (without the compound added) as well as compound controls (without virus).

5. Incubate the plates for 48–72 h in 5% CO_2 in air. Fix, stain, dry, and count plaques as described before (*Protocol 2*).

6. The mean plaque counts in wells exposed to the compound are calculated and related to the plaque count in wells without the compound. The effect of the compound at different concentrations is expressed in terms of % plaques of seeded plaque count or % reduction in seeded plaque count. The IC_{50} is determined as the concentration of compound giving a 50% reduction in the plaque count of the inoculum (*Figure 3*).

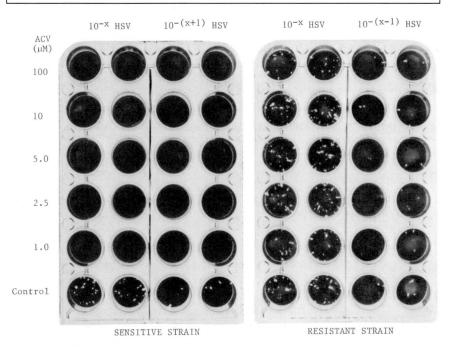

Figure 2. Results of plaque reduction assays with herpes simplex virus (HSV) isolates either resistant or sensitive to acyclovir (ACV).

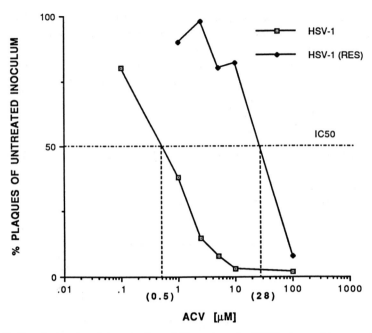

Figure 3. Graph showing determination of IC_{50} values for HSV isolates either sensitive or resistant to acyclovir.

4.2 Colorimetric assays

The formazan assay system is used and has been described in detail in *Protocol 4* (reference 10).

Protocol 7. Colorimetric assay for evaluating anti-HIV agents in acutely infected cells.

1. Prepare cultures of permissive cells (e.g. C8166 or MT4) in 96-well plates (*Figure 4*).

2. Infect half the cells with HIV (100 $TCID_{50}$ per well) in the presence of a dilution series of the antiviral compound(s) to be tested and proceed as before.

3. Arrange the samples so that, for each compound, infected and un-infected cells and treated and untreated cells, are adjacent (*Figure 4*). Compare the cut-off points and then measure the optical density on a plate reader.

4. Calculate the percent inhibition achieved by the compounds using the following formula:

$$\frac{(OD_T)_{HIV} - (OD_C)_{HIV}}{(OD_C)_{mock} - (OD_C)_{HIV}} \times 100$$

---

in which $(OD_T)_{HIV}$ is the optical density measured at a given concentration of compound with HIV-infected cells; $(OD_C)_{HIV}$ is the optical density measured for the untreated control HIV-infected cells; $(OD_C)_{mock}$ is the optical density measured for the untreated control mock infected cells. Plot the CD_{50} and the IC_{50} values against concentration on the same graph and compare the antiviral effect and toxicity properties of the compound directly (*Figure 5*).

4.3 Antiviral array using HIV-1 p24 antigen production

Protocol 8 describes another method for assaying the efficacy of antiviral agents. The p24 antigen is measured with a commercially available enzyme

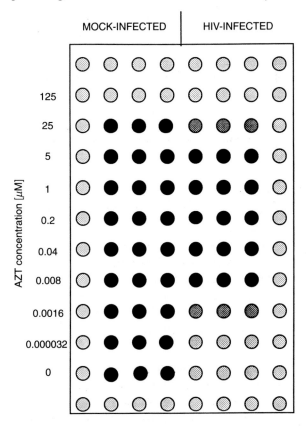

Figure 4. Diagram of microtitre plate illustrating the MTT procedure. Viable wells are shown as black, no growth is shown as white, and intermediate growth is indicated by shading. The middle three rows on the left are mock-infected; the middle three rows on the right are HIV-infected cells. All wells are exposed to varying concentrations of AZT. The outside wells contain medium only. (From ref. 19; reprinted with the permission of Elsevier Science Publishers.)

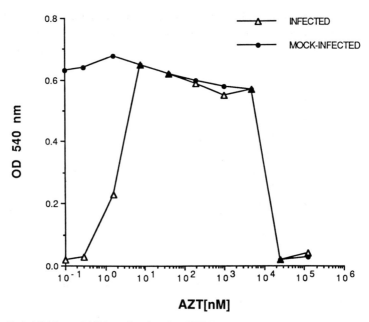

Figure 5. Inhibition of HIV replication by AZT in cell suspensions in the MTT assay. AZT (●) is active at low concentration and its toxic effect (△) is observed at higher concentrations.

immuno-assay (EIA). These kits give results which are highly reproducible from one assay to another and are useful when evaluating structure–activity relationships between closely related compounds. Usually sample volumes of 1.5 ml are used in assays in 6 ml tubes; this eliminates the 'edge effects' that may occur with smaller volumes in plate systems. In practice the maximum number of tubes that can be manipulated at any one time is 150. However, this assay system is easily adapted to a 96-well format, in which case culture volumes and the number of cells are divided by 10. The 96-well format may have to be used if only small amounts of compounds (<1 mg) are available for testing.

Protocol 8. Antiviral assay using p24 antigen production as a marker for HIV replication in acutely infected cells

1. Establish the number of sample tubes (duplicates) needed for the assay and hence the total number of cells required. Split the cells on the day prior to the assay so that they will be in log phase of replication at the start of the assay. Count the concentration of cells in the stock culture with a haemocytometer and centrifuge the necessary volume of stock culture in a universal container in a bench-top centrifuge (1100 r.p.m. for 5 min).

---

2. Remove the culture medium, break up the pellet by flicking the universal container, and add the appropriate volume of HIV virus stock (containing 10 $TCID_{50}$) per 2×10^5 cells. Transfer the mixture to a 50 cm^2 culture flask and ensure that the cells are evenly distributed in the supernatant. Incubate the cells in 5% CO_2 in air at 37 °C for 1.5 h.

3. Wash the infected cells three times in a universal container with 20 ml of PBS to remove unadsorbed virus.

4. Resuspend aliquots of 2×10^5 cells in 1.5 ml of growth medium in the presence of each compound at serial log or half log dilution steps and incubate at 37 °C for 72 h in 5% CO_2 in air. Compounds are dissolved in water, DMSO, or occasionally in other solvents such as ethanol. Drug dilutions are carried out in growth medium using a programmable dispenser which achieves high reproducibility of pipetting. AZT (0.001– 1 μM) and dideoxycytidine (ddC) (0.03–10 μM) can be included as internal controls when testing novel compounds, together with both uninfected and infected untreated cells.

5. Take 100 μl samples from each tube and measure the HIV p24 antigen in the supernatants using a commercial EIA following the manufacturer's protocol (11).

6. Plot a curve of optical density at 450 nm (OD_{450}) against concentration for each compound. Draw the '50% line' (half the average OD_{450} value for the infected untreated control) and plot the IC_{50} value for each compound (*Figure 6*).

4.4 Assays with cells chronically infected with HIV

Chronically infected cells can be used to evaluate the activity of those compounds which act on post-integration events such as gene expression or release of virus from cells (*Protocol 9*).

Protocol 9. Assays with cells chronically infected with HIV

1. Count the concentration of chronically infected cells (e.g. $H9_{RF}$) in the stock culture with a haemocytometer and centrifuge (1100 r.p.m. for 5 min) the necessary volume (10^4 cells per well) of stock culture in a universal container. Wash the cells twice in PBS (20 ml) to remove free virus.

2. Resuspend the cells in growth medium (RPMI 1640 plus 10% fetal bovine serum) and pipette 200 μl volumes containing 10^4 cells into each well.

3. Add the compounds in the appropriate log or half log dilution series.

Protocol 9. *Continued*

4. Withdraw 100 µl samples of the supernatants from treated and untreated wells after 72–96 h and test for p24 antigen production as
described in (*Protocol 8*).

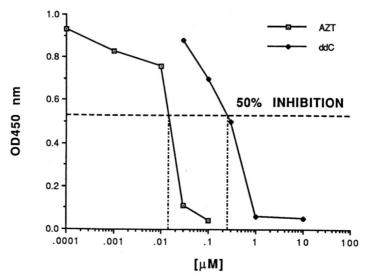

Figure 6. Comparison of the activity of AZT and ddC in the antigen reduction asay.
Neither of these compounds is toxic at 100 µM in this assay system.

4.5 Back titration assays

These assay systems can be used in conjunction with other systems (see
Sections 4.3 and 4.4) in order to evaluate compounds which act at late stages
of virus replication and thus may lead to the release of non-infectious virus
particles. Supernatants from the primary cultures, containing different concentrations of the drug, are titrated on to indicator cells and the development
of CPE in the indicator cells is assessed as a measure of the antiviral activity.
C8166 and CEM cells form syncytia readily, but MT2, MT4 and JM cells form
syncytia which are more distinctive and easier to count. Thus the latter may
be more suitable as indicator cells for use in these assays.

Protocol 10. Back titration assay

1. Seed the wells of a 96-well plate with uninfected indicator cells: 2×10^4
cells per 100 µl fresh culture medium per well.

2. Titrate, by serial dilutions, the supernatants of each well (or tubes) of

the primary cultures, containing different concentrations of com-pounds, on to the indicator cells (e.g. doubling dilutions, log or half log intervals). Make sure that each well finally contains 200 μl of medium.

3. Inspect the plate each day and score the formation of syncytia, either on a semi-quantitative basis ($+++/++/+/-$) or by counting individual syncytia. The infectivity in the original inoculum and hence the effect of the antiviral compound is assessed by inhibition of CPE.

4.6 Pre-treatment of cells or virus

Compounds which effect binding and uncoating may not show any activity unless added to the cells a few hours before infection. If dose-response curves are required then uninfected cell aliquots are treated, either in plates or tubes, with compounds at various dilutions 1–24 h before infection. Each cell aliquot is infected with the appropriate volume of virus supernatant (e.g. 10 $TCID_{50}$). For evaluation by antigen capture it is necessary to wash each sample after 1.5 h and then add fresh compound. For the formazan assay and those assays which use CPE as an end-point the intermediate washing step may be omitted, although it may be necessary to use a lower multiplicity of infection in these assays than previously. To assess the direct antiviral effect of a compound, the virus stock is treated with the compound (using an appropriate dilution series) before addition to the cells.

4.7 Mixed cell assays for HIV

This method is used to test the effect of compounds, such as soluble CD^+, which bind to gp120 expressed on chronically infected cells. Similarly, the effect of compounds which block $CD4^+$ on uninfected T-lymphoblasts may be assessed. Thus, chronically infected cells and uninfected $CD4^+$ cells are mixed and the antiviral effects are measured by the inhibition of CPE.

Protocol 11. Mixed cell assays for HIV

1. Pre-incubate either chronically infected cells (e.g. H9$_{RF}$), or CD4$^+$ cells (e.g. C8166 or MT4) with the compound, in the appropriate log or half log dilution series, for a minimum of 2 h (preferably overnight).

2. Before mixing the two cell types, wash and resuspend the chronically infected cells twice in PBS to remove the supernatant containing HIV. If the chronically infected cells have been pre-treated, resuspend them in the medium containing the appropriate dilutions of compound. The washing procedure is to ensure that compounds are given the best chance to show activity in the assay but washing may be omitted and cells mixed immediately after pre-incubation.

Protocol 11. *Continued*

3. Resuspend the two cell types mixed together in growth medium at a ratio of 1:10 of infected: uninfected cells. If 96-well plates are used then resuspend 10^4 mixed cells in 200 μl; if 24-well plates or 6 ml tubes are used then resupend 2×10^5 cells in 1.5 ml. These ratios may be changed to modify the sensitivity of the assay.

4. Sample the supernatants after 96 h and count syncytia.

4.8 Delayed addition experiments

With all the methods outlined above the compounds can be added at various times post-infection in order to investigate the stage at which new compounds act. The end-points are determined simultaneously at the appropriate time so that the total incubation period becomes uniform. Usually these experiments are carried out with concentrations of compounds 10–100 times higher than the IC_{50} values. This pre-supposes that no toxic effects are observed at the concentrations used. The activity of novel compounds should be tested in parallel with those of known activity so that the stage in the replication cycle of the virus can be established. The replication time for the virus can be compared with the time at which compound efficacy is lost, thus indicating which step the compound is inhibiting. Alternatively, it may be possible to test the cultures for accumulation of viral gene products, such as early or late antigens, produced prior to the blocked stage.

4.9 Combination studies

The ability of viruses to develop resistance to currently available antiviral agents has been demonstrated by culture of viruses in the presence of drugs *in vitro* and by observation of infections *in vivo* which appear to be resistant to chemotherapy and from which resistant viruses have been isolated. The phenomenon of emerging drug resistance of herpesviruses and HIV has been seen mainly in the most heavily immunocompromised individuals and is thought to be related to increased levels of virus replication.

A major reason for considering the use of combination therapy is to attempt to inhibit the emergence of a resistant sub-population of virus by inhibiting the viral replication cycle at two or more distinct target sites. The value of combination therapy over monotherapy has been proven in anti-bacterial strategies, particularly in the treatment of tuberculosis. Another important potential benefit of the use of combination therapy results from the existence of synergistic activity of some drug combinations. If synergy can be shown to occur, effective antiviral activity will be achieved with reduced doses of the individual drugs. It may therefore be possible to reduce or remove the danger of toxic side effects while maintaining adequate control of the infection. Even if a combination is only additive in its activity, the summation of the effects of two or more drugs will mean that lower doses of each component will be required, thus reducing the risks of toxicity.

The *in vitro* evaluation of two or more compounds in combination may be investigated by the techniques described in previous sections; however, interpretation of the data may be difficult when deciding between additive and synergistic effects. The theoretical principles and practical examples of a large number of antiviral combinations are reviewed in reference 12. Combination studies would normally only be carried out with compounds which have shown a good antiviral activity in tissue culture, thus it is imperative to have consistent IC_{50} and cytotoxicity values for each compound in question. Furthermore, cytotoxicity of the compound combination should be determined in uninfected cells before proceeding to the antiviral studies. The following notes describe the approach to evaluating agents in combination against HIV.

(a) Select a concentration range for each compound that is at least two logs above and below the IC_{50} values for each compound. The concentrations used should be two-to five-fold serial dilutions from the highest concentrations used (13). The dilutions may depend upon the software chosen for analysis of the results since some programmes are more flexible in their requirements for intervals. The solubility of the compound may also be a limiting factor in reaching the highest concentration.

(b) Evaluate the toxicity, as described in Section 3, of the compound combination in the format of a chequer-board titration.

(c) If the compounds show no additive effects in their toxicity then follow the methods described above for assaying antiviral activity. A chequer-board arrangement of concentrations is set up with the appropriate controls and p24 antigen or formazan production can be measured as described previously (see *Protocols 7* and *8*).

(d) Semi-quantitative values can be deduced from the measurements of p24 antigen data (or CPE) and the determination of synergy can be demonstrated by construction of isobolograms. The analysis of the results can be assisted by the use of PC programs (14) or with the Macintosh system (MacSynergy).

5. Activity against isolated viral enzymes

For antiviral compounds targeted against specific viral enzymes it may be possible to study the activity directly on preparations of the enzymes. Thus extensive studies have been carried out on herpesvirus thymidine kinase (TK) and polymerase, and on HIV reverse transcriptase. The following sections describe some of the methods used for the preparation and study of viral enzymes.

In enzyme-catalysed reactions, some of the binding energy between the enzyme and the substrate contributes directly to the catalysis so that, as the substrate molecules pass through a series of intermediate forms, the free energies of the most unstable transition states are greatly reduced, and consequently greatly accelerate these reactions. For most enzymes, the concentration of substrate (in μM) at which the reaction rate is half-maximal (i.e. when half the binding sites are occupied) is a measure of how tightly a particular substrate and enzyme are bound together. This concentration is known as the Michaelis constant (K_M). Thus a low value for K_M indicates strong binding, and for most single substrate enzymatic reactions the value for K_M is between 10^{-5} and 10^{-2} M.

For competitive inhibition to occur, the antiviral agent needs to bind to the enzyme in the site normally occupied by the substrate. The extent of this inhibition is related to the concentrations of the inhibitor and the substrate. The binding of inhibitor to enzyme is usually reversible; the dissociation of the inhibitor–enzyme complex is measured in μM and is called the dissociation constant (K_i). This value should be low for the inhibitor–virus enzyme complex (indicating a high affinity), but high (indicating low affinity) for cellular enzymes. *Table 3* shows examples of K_i values for some nucleoside analogues with viral and cellular enzymes. Mutations in the viral enzyme which lead to drug resistance manifest as a reduction in the affinity of the inhibitor–enzyme complex, which is indicated by an increase in the K_i value (*Table 3*). Such mutations do not necessarily affect the normal functions of the enzyme. The underlying mechanisms of selectivity at the level of the enzymes are still poorly understood. It is not clear, for example, how HSV TK recognizes analogues such as ACV and then phosphorylates them. Some analogues, such as 5-bromodeoxyuridine, are readily recognized by HSV-1 TK but poorly phosphorylated by HSV-2 TK. Preparations of purified enzymes for studies on inhibitors may be obtained either from infected cells or from recombinant DNA products.

To establish the potency and selectivity of compounds, they are tested

---

Table 3. Kinetic values for substrates and inhibitors of cellular and viral enzymes

Enzyme	Substrate	K_m (μM)	Analogue	K_i (μM)
HSV pol	dGTP	0.7	ACV-TP	0.015
HSV TK	Thymidine	0.2	ACV	200
HSV TKR	Thymidine	2.5	ACV	2500
Cellular TK	Thymidine	1.3	ACV	>250
HIV RT	dTTP	0.3	AZT-TP	0.01
H9 pol	dTTP	2.4	AZT-TP	230

pol = DNA polymerase; TK = thymidine kinase; ACV = acyclovir; AZT = azidothymidine; TP = triphosphate; dTTP = deoxy thymidine triphosphate; TKR = TK resistant

---

against both the viral target enzymes and related cellular enzymes. For inhibitors of viral polymerases, compounds are tested also against cellular DNA polymerases; for inhibitors of HIV proteinase, compounds are tested against cellular proteinases.

The conditions for enzyme extraction have been optimized for each of the two methods described (*Protocols 12* and *13*). Essentially each method requires a phosphate buffer (pH range from 7.5 to 8.3) in the presence of reducing agents, such as DTT. Glycerol is included to assist in loading the preparation on to columns.

An assay for HIV reverse transcriptase and its inhibition is described in *Protocol 14*, and for cellular polymerases and their inhibition in *Protocol 15*, *Protocol 16* contains an assay for measuring HIV proteinase and its inhibition.

Protocol 12. Preparation of reverse transcriptase from HIV-infected cells

The method of Chandra *et al.* (reference 15) is followed and is generally applicable for viral polymerases.

1. Centrifuge 10^8–10^9 H9 cells, chronically infected with HIV, in a universal container at 1100 r.p.m. for 10 min. Remove the supernatant and add 3 ml of a buffer containing 1% (w/v) SDS and 1% (w/v) Triton X-100 in 10 mM Tris–HCl (pH 8.3). Vortex the mixture thoroughly and leave at room temperature for 30 min.

2. Dialyse the lysate against 10 mM Tris–HCl (pH 8.3) containing 1 mM DTT and 10% glycerol, and apply it to a sephacryl S-400 HR column (Pharmacia) equilibrated with the same buffer.

3. Elute the column with a gradient of 10 mM Tris–HCl (pH 8.3), to 50 mM Tris–HCl (pH 7.9) with 0.3 M KCl, 1 mM DTT, and 10% glycerol. The elution of protein is monitored at 280 nm and, unless it is known which fraction contains the enzyme, it will be necessary to test all protein-containing fractions for activity.

4. Dialyse the eluent containing the enzyme against 10 mM Tris–HCl (pH 7.5), 1 mM DTT, and 10% glycerol and apply to a phosphocellulose column (P-11, Pharmacia) equilibrated with the same buffer.

5. Elute the column with a gradient of 10 mM Tris–HCl (pH 7.5) to 50 mM Tris–HCl (pH 7.9) with 0.7 M KCl, 1 mM DTT and 10% glycerol. Monitor protein peaks at 280 nm and test for RT activity (*Protocol 14*).

6. Dialyse the purified enzyme against 20 mM Tris-HCl (pH 7.5), 1 mM DTT, and 10% glycerol. Concentrate the enzyme preparation in an Amicon ultrafiltration cell and store at −70 °C until needed.

Protocol 13. Preparation of HIV reverse transcriptase from *Escherichia coli* containing a recombinant plasmid

The method of Le Grise *et al.* (reference 16) is followed and is generally applicable for recombinant plasmids containing polymerases.

1. Grow the recombinant plasmid, (e.g. pRt/I10) containing a functional HIV reverse transcriptase gene, in *E. coli* and induce expression with isopropyl-β-D-thiogalactopyranoside (IPTG) (400 μg/ml) overnight.

2. Harvest cells by centrifugation (6000 r.p.m. for 15 min at 4 °C). Resuspend cells in 2 ml lysozyme (1 mg/ml in 0.25 M Na_2EDTA, pH 8) for 5 min and then treat with 1 mg/ml DNase 1 for 1 h at 37 °C.

3. Centrifuge the lysate at 5000 g for 30 min at 4 °C, recover the supernatant and add solid ammonium sulphate to 55% (w/v).

4. Leave for 1 h on ice and then collect the precipitate by centrifugation and dissolve in buffer containing 50 mM Tris–HCl (pH 7.9), 1 mM DTT, and 10% glycerol.

5. Purify the crude HIV-1 RT preparation further by passing it through a Sephacryl S-400 HR column pre-equilibrated with the same buffer as above (*Protocol 12*) and collect the enriched HIV-1 RT eluent.

Protocol 14. Assay for HIV reverse transcriptase and its inhibition by measuring the incorporation of tritiated dNTP

This method is generally applicable to other DNA polymerases with the appropriate modifications.

1. Place 10–20 μl of the purified enzyme preparation on ice.

2. Adjust the buffer to give final concentrations of 50 mM Tris–HCl (pH 7.9), 1 mM DTT, 5 mM $MgCl_2$, 50 mM KCl, and 0.25 units/ml of poly(A)(dT)$_{15}$ primer if the inhibitors are analogues of thymidine. For analogues of cytidine, guanosine, or adenine the appropriate template primer system must be used.

3. Add inhibitors (5–10 μl volumes) at a series of concentrations (e.g. 0.001–10 μM) to the buffered enzyme.

4. Add 10 μl of tritiated thymidine triphosphate ([^{3}H]TTP) in water (1 μCi) and then add sterile water to give a final volume of 100 μl. Incubate in a shaking water bath at 37 °C for 1–2 h.

5. Stop the reactions by adding an equal volume of 20% ice-cold trichloroacetic acid (TCA) and keep the mixtures cold for 1 h.

6. Collect precipitates on Whatman GF/B filters in a manifold (Millipore) and wash with ice-cold 10% TCA (3 × 5 ml) and, finally, once with absolute alcohol.

7. Air-dry the filters or use an oven at 37 °C and process the filters for β-scintillation counting.

Protocol 15. Assay of compounds against cellular polymerases to determine the selectivity of nucleoside analogues

The calculation of the selectivity of AZT against HIV-1 reverse transcriptase is summarized in *Table 4* as an example.

1. Extract α and γ polymerases from HeLa cells (2 ml packed cell volume) by brief sonication in five volumes of buffer containing 300 mM K_2PO_4 (pH 7.5) 0.1% NP40, 1 mM EDTA, 1 mM DTT, and 10% glycerol.

2. Purify the enzymes by DE-52 cellulose and phosphocellulose column chromatography as described in *Protocol 12*.

3. Place 10–20 µl of the enzyme preparation on ice and add 50 mM Tris–HCl (pH 8), 0.5 mM DTT, 50 µg/ml bovine serum albumin (BSA), and 125 µg/ml activated salmon sperm or calf thymus DNA. In addition the reaction mixture should contain either 8 mM $MgCl_2$ for assays of α polymerase, or 0.5 mM $MnCl_2$, 100 mM KCl, and 50 mM K_2PO_4 (pH 8) for γ polymerase.

4. Add dilutions of the inhibitors followed by dATP, dGTP, dCTP, and [^{3}H]dTTP. If [^{3}H]dCTP is used as the label then omit the cold dCTP but add dTTP. Add sterile water to give a final reaction volume of 100 µl.

5. Incubate and count the incorporated radiolabel as described in *Protocol 14.*

Table 4. Selectivity of AZT against HIV-1 reverse transcriptase

Enzyme	Template	K_M for TTP (µM)	K_i for AZTTP (µM)	Affinity ratio (K_M/K_i)	Selectivity index [a]
α-polymerase	Gapped DNA	7.8	>100	<0.08	>50
β-polymerase	Gapped DNA	1.3	100	0.013	308
γ-polymerase	Gapped DNA	0.1	22	0.0045	889
HIV RT	Gapped DNA	1.2	0.3	4	–

[a] Selectivity index = $\dfrac{\text{HIV-1 RT } K_m/K_i}{\text{polymerase } K_M/K_i}$

Protocol 16. Assay for HIV proteinase and inhibitors

The colorimetric assay method of Broadhurst *et al.* (18) is used to measure the activity of small protected peptides as inhibitors of HIV proteinase (5). Synthetic substrates of HIV proteinase are cleaved by the enzyme to release N-terminal propyl peptides which react with isatin to form a blue product which is measured spectroscopically. The assay is suitable for use with pure enzyme or crude extracts derived from genetically engineered plasmids grown in *Escherichia coli.*

1. Prepare crude HIV-1 proteinase from *E. coli* pTAN by using the procedure described in *Protocol 13* (see also reference 17).

2. Dissolve the peptide substrate (0.5–0.7 mM depending upon molecular weight) in 125 mM sodium citrate (pH 5.5) and 0.0125% Tween 20. A heptapeptide substrate has been chosen for routine use in the assay as it gives the assay maximal sensitivity (18).

3. Incubate 80 μl of the buffered substrate plus proteinase (see *Protocol 13*) and a synthetic peptide inhibitor (0.0001–1 μM depending upon activity; e.g. R031–8959) in a reaction volume of 100 μl at 37 °C in 15 × 85 mm borosilicate glass tubes for 30 min.

4. Stop the reaction by adding 1 ml of the colour reagent (isatin (Sigma), 30 μg/ml), and 2-(4-chlorobenzoyl)benzoic acid (1.5 mg/ml) in 10% acetone in ethanol.

5. Immerse the uncovered tubes in a boiling water bath to a depth of 3 cm for 15 min, and evaporate the solvent to leave a pigmented residue.

6. Cool to room temperature and add 1 ml of a solution of 1% pyrogallol in acetone:water (2:1) to dissolve the pigment. This should be carried out away from direct sunlight as the blue pigment is light-sensitive.

7. Measure the optical density immediately at 599 nm and plot optical density against concentration.

References

1. Bauer, D. J., St Vincent, L., Kempe, C. H., and Downie, A. W. (1963). *Lancet,* **ii**, 494.
2. Elion, G. B., Furman, P. A., Fyfe, J. A., de Miranda, P., Beauchamp, I., and Schaeffer, H. J. (1977). *Proc. Natl. Acad. Sci. USA,* **74**, 5716.
3. Mar, E. C., Cheng, Y. C., and Huang, E. S. (1983). *Antimicrob. Agents Chemother.,* **24**, 518.
4. Mitsuya, H., *et al.* (1985). *Proc. Natl. Acad. Sci. USA,* **82**, 7096.
5. Roberts, N. A., Martin, J. A., Kinchington, D., Broadhurst, A. V., Duncan, I. B., Galpin, S. A., *et al.* (1990). *Science,* **248**, 358.

6. Belshe, R. B., Hall-Smith, M., Hall C. B., Betts, R., and Hay, A. J. (1988). *J. Virol.*, **62**, 1508.
7. Rossmann, M. G., Arnold, E., Erickson, J. W., *et al.* (1985). *Nature* (London) **317**, 145.
8. Smith, T. J., Kremer, M. J., Luo, M., *et al.* (1986). *Science*, **233**, 1286.
9. Dulbecco, R. (1988). *Virology*, 2nd edn, pp. 22–5. J. P. Lippincott, Philadelphia.
10. Pauwels, R., Balzarini, J., Baba, M., Snoeck, R., Schols, D., Herdewijn, D. P., Desmyter, J., and De Clercq, E. (1988). *J. Virol. Methods*, **20**, 309.
11. Kinchington, D., Galpin, S. A., O'Connor, T. J., Jeffries, D. J., and Williamson, J. D. (1989). *AIDS*, **3**, 101.
12. Hall, M. J. and Duncan, I. B. (1987). In *Antiviral agents* (ed. H. J. Field). CRC Press, Boca Raton, FL.
13. Johnston, V. A. (1990). In *Techniques in HIV research* (ed. A. Aldovini and B. D. Walker), pp. 232–7. Stockton Press, USA.
14. Chou, J. and Talay, T. C. (1987). *A computer software for IBM-PC and manual.* Elsevier-Biosoft, Cambridge, UK.
15. Chandra, P., Vogel, A., and Gerber, T. (1985). *Cancer Res.*, **45**, 4677.
16. Le Grise, S. F., Zehnle, R., and Mous, J. (1988). *J. Virol.*, **62**, 2525.
17. Graves, M. C., Meidal, M. C., Pan, Y. C. E., Manneberg, M., Lahm, H. W., and Gruninger-Leitch, R. (1990). *Biochem. Biophys. Res. Commun.*, **168**, 30.
18. Broadhurst, A. V., Roberts, N. A., Ritchie, A. J., Handa B. K., and Kay, C. (1991). *Anal. Biochem.*, **193**, 280.

7

Molecular epidemiology

U. DESSELBERGER

1. Introduction

Knowledge of the epidemiology of infectious diseases is much older than the recognition of their causative agents. Transmission modes, vectors, point sources, seasonality, etc., were known long before the first micro-organisms were recognized as causing infectious disease according to Koch's criteria. For viruses this was established just 100 years ago, and their identification as pathogenic agents is not complete even now (1).

Viruses are classified, according to their physical structure and to replication strategies, into families, subfamilies, and genera. The development of immunology allowed further subdivision into types, subtypes, and strains according to differences in the antigenic composition of physically identical particles, and in the 1950s and 1960s much was learned about the serological classification of viruses causing outbreaks and epidemics, e.g., the linkage of the appearance of new influenza A virus subtypes with pandemics of influenza, or of poliovirus types with outbreaks of paralytic disease. Serology also confirmed that certain viruses causing epidemics seemed to be 'monotypic' (e.g. measles virus and rubella virus).

The advent of methods to analyse viruses at the molecular level, particularly of methods to analyse the genome, has added a plethora of additional parameters of virus characterization which have been extensively used for correlation with epidemiological data. Thus the term 'molecular epidemiology' was coined to denote the use of biochemical and molecular techniques to investigate and complement viral epidemiology. There are recent examples that show that molecular techniques are a necessary prerequisite to establish the epidemiology of viral infections.

Some molecular techniques are described below and examples of their application to epidemiological analysis given. No completeness is claimed, as the field of molecular virology is rapidly developing and epidemiological applications are following fast. Many of the techniques are described in great detail in Sambrook et al. (2).

The analyses describe here relate to pieces of genomic nucleic acid (RNA segments, RNA oligonucleotides, and DNA fragments), or to nucleotide and predicted amino acid sequences obtained by cloning and sequencing or by direct sequencing techniques.

2. Use of polyacrylamide gel electrophoresis to separate the segments of RNA viruses

When it became known that the genome of some RNA viruses consisted of separate entities called segments which are separately replicated and then assorted into progeny virus particles and which can be easily purified and separated by PAGE, this procedure was applied to analyse the genomes of viral isolates obtained during outbreaks and epidemics. *Protocol 1* describes the extraction of viral RNA, *Protocol 2* electrophoresis, and *Protocol 3* staining of gels containing separated RNA segments.

Protocol 1. Extraction of viral RNA (e.g. human rotavirus RNA)

A. *Preparation of virus sample*

1. Make a 20% suspension of human faeces in PBS (0.15 M NaCl in 0.01 M phosphate, pH 7.4) and mix.
2. Centrifuge at 1500 g for 5 min at room temperature.
3. Overlay supernatant (e.g. 5 ml) on to a cushion of 0.5 ml of 30% sucrose (in PBS) in ultracentrifuge tube.
4. Ultracentrifuge in swing-out bucket rotor at 60 000 g for 1 h at 15 °C.
5. Discard supernatant and resuspend pellet in 0.1 ml PBS (= virus sample).

B. *RNA extraction*

6. Dilute 50 µl of virus sample with 200 µl of 0.25 M NaCl containing 1% (w/v) SDS in an Eppendorf tube.
7. Mix with one volume of phenol/chloroform (1:1, w/w equilibrated with 0.25 M NaCl); keep at 56 °C for 10 min with repeated mixing.
8. Spin at 11 000 g for 5 min at room temperature.
9. Remove (aqueous) supernatant (upper phase) and repeat steps 7 and 8 until interphase is clear.
10. Extract aqueous phase twice with ether (note: the aqueous phase is the lower phase). The phases separate quickly, so no centrifugation is necessary.
11. Precipitate RNA from aqueous phase by adding 2.5 volumes of ethanol. Mix. Keep at −70 °C for 20 min.
12. Thaw, mix, and centrifuge at 11 000 g for 10 min.

---

13. Remove supernatant, dry pellet in freeze drier or vacufuge, and re-dissolve in 10–20 μl of TE buffer (0.01 M Tris–HCl, pH 7.4, 1 mM EDTA) (=RNA sample).

Protocol 2. Polyacrylamide gel electrophoresis of viral RNA

1. Clean two glass plates (20 × 20 cm or bigger; one plain and one notched) with 70% ethanol and ether. Arrange 1 mm thick spacers at each side parallel to the edges and bind the sides and bottom of plates with gel-sealing tape.

2. Prepare 10% resolving gel consisting of:
- 30% acrylamide-*bis* (29% acrylamide, 1% *N,N'*-methylene-*bis*-acrylamide)   16.6 ml
- 1.5 M Tris–HCl, pH 8.8   12.5 ml
- *N,N,N',N'*-tetramethylene diamine (TEMED)   12 μl
- 20% ammonium persulphate (APS, freshly prepared, in water)   600 μl
- de-ionized water   20.3 ml
                                                                                (Total 50.0 ml)

Pour an 18 × 15 cm gel between plates, overlay with a 3 mm layer of water-saturated butanol, and allow to polymerize (1 h).

3. Remove butanol, wash gel with distilled water, and overlay with 3% stacking gel consisting of
- 30% acrylamide–*bis*-acrylamide   1.0 ml
- 0.5 M Tris–HCl, pH 6.8   2.5 ml
- TEMED   10 μl
- 20% APS   200 μl
- de-ionized water   6.3 ml
                                                                                (Total 10.0 ml)

Insert comb (1 mm thick), clamp top with metal clip, and allow to polymerize (30 min).

4. Remove comb, wash slots carefully with distilled water, and overlay with running buffer containing
- 25 mM Tris–HCl pH 8.3
- 192 mM glycine

Attach gel to electrophoresis tank, prerun at 5 mA for 1 h.

5. Mix one volume of RNA sample, approximately 5 μl, with one volume of running mix containing:
- 2 × running buffer
- 20% sucrose

Protocol 2. *Continued*

- 0.1% bromophenol blue
- 0.1% xylene cyanol FF

6. Load specimens into slots and electrophorese at 15 mA for 16–20 h.

7. Remove one plate and fix gel with 10% ethanol/5% glacial acetic acid in water for 1 h prior to silver staining (see *Protocol 3*).

Protocol 3. Staining of viral RNA segments in polyacrylamide gels

A. *Staining with ethidium bromide*

1. Add ethidium bromide to the gel and running buffer at a concentration of 0.5 μg/ml.

2. Examine under UV illumination.

B. *Staining with silver*

1. Immerse fixed gel (on plate) (*Protocol 2*, step 7) in 0.19% silver nitrate solution for 30 min.

2. Remove excess silver nitrate by rinsing three times with tap water.

3. Treat gel for 5–10 min with reducing solution consisting of
   - sodium borohydride 0.01% (w/v)
   - sodium hydroxide 3.0% (w/v)
   - formaldehyde 0.3% (w/v)

   until RNA segments become visible.

4. Immerse gel in 5% ethanol, 5% acetic acid (according to Whitton *et al.* (3)).

The method has been extensively used to describe 'electropherotypes' of rotaviruses (4–8). It was generally found that different electropherotypes co-circulated during winter outbreaks of rotavirus infections. The method was sufficiently precise to state that close outbreaks, e.g. those in hospitals, were due to a virus of identical electropherotype, but it was soon realized that viruses of the same serotype (determined by neutralizing antibodies) showed different electropherotypes (6, 8), and, vice versa, that viruses of indistinguishable electropherotype belonged to different serotypes (9). Therefore the epidemiological value of electropherotyping decreased in favour of serotyping. On the other hand, electropherotyping of rotaviruses has led to the detection of genome rearrangements (7, 10).

3. Oligonucleotide maps of RNA virus genomes

Digestion of denatured viral RNA with certain ribonucleases (RNases) yields oligonucleotides of unique composition. RNase T1 cuts only after G residues resulting in oligonucleotides with free 5'-end hydroxyl group and 3'-end guanosine monophosphate residues. After phosphatase treatment (to remove 5' terminal phosphate of RNA) oligonucleotides can be labelled using $[\gamma\text{-}^{32}P]ATP$ and polynucleotide kinase, and the labelled oligonucleotides can be separated by two-dimensional (2D) PAGE followed by autoradiography. *Protocol 4* describes the preparation of labelled oligonucleotides and *Protocol 5* the 2D PAGE.

Protocol 4. RNase T1 digestion of viral RNA and radiolabelling of resulting oligonucleotides

1. In an Eppendorf tube, mix
   - 1 μl of viral RNA (1 μg) in 20 mM Tris–HCl pH 8.0, 2 mM EDTA
   - 1 μl of RNase T1 (Sankyo, Calbiochem, 1 unit) in same buffer
   - 1 μl of calf intestine alkaline phosphatase (New England Biolabs) (10^{-2} units)

   and incubate for 60 min at 37 °C.

2. (a) Add 50 μl of polynucleotide kinase reaction mixture containing:
   - 10 mM KH_2PO_4/K_3PO_4, pH 9.5
   - 10 mM $Mg(OAc)_2$
   - 5 mM dithiothreitol (DTT)
   - 50 μCi of $[\gamma\text{-}^{32}P]$ ATP (sp. act. 3000 Ci/mmol)
   - polynucleotide kinase (New England Biolabs or P-L Biochemicals, 2 units)

   (b) Incubate for 3–16 h at 37 °C.

3. Add 50 μl of 0.6 M $NH_4(OAc)$ containing 50 μg of yeast tRNA (carrier).

4. Extract with 100 μl of phenol (saturated with 10 mM Tris–HCl, pH 8) at room temperature.

5. Repeat step 4 twice until the interface is clear.

6. Mix aqueous phase with 300 μl of 95% ethanol and keep at −70 °C for 30 min.

7. Pellet oligonucleotides at 11 000 g for 10 min at room temperature.

8. Freeze-dry pellet and dissolve in 10 μl of running solution containing
   - 10 mM citrate pH 5.0
   - 1 mM EDTA
   - 7 M urea
   - 0.1% bromophenol blue
   - 0.1% xylene cyanol FF
   - 200 μg/ml yeast tRNA (carrier)

Protocol 5. Two dimensional PAGE of radiolabelled RNase T1-resistant oligonucleotides

1. Gel glass plates measuring 40 × 20 × 0.3 cm are put together as described in *Protocol 2*. Spacers of 1 mm thickness are used.

2. (a) Make gel solution of the following composition:
   - 10% acrylamide
   - 0.3% *N,N'*-methylene bisacrylamide
   - 0.025 M citric acid, pH 3.5
   - 6 M urea (ultrapure, Schwarz Mann)
   (b) Filter through 0.45 μm filter (Millipore) before pouring.
   (c) Start polymerization by adding (per 100 ml)
   - 0.4 ml of $FeSO_4 \cdot 7H_2O$ (2.5 mg/ml, fresh)
   - 0.4 ml ascorbic acid (100 mg/ml, fresh)
   - 0.04 ml of 30% H_2O_2

3. Mix and pour between gel plates. Insert comb (with six to eight slots, 5 × 10 mm) and press between glass plates using paper clips. Wait 30 min for polymerization to occur.

4. Place plates in tank filled with 6 litres of 0.025 M citric acid and connect top by a paper wick with another tank containing 4 litres of 0.025 M citric acid.

5. Pre-electrophorese at 1000 V for 20 min.

6. Rinse slots and apply 5–10 μl of 5'-^{32}P-labelled oligonucleotides.

7. Electrophorese (in a 4 °C room) at 1700 V (at approximately 30 mA) until bromophenol blue has moved 20 cm.

8. Remove one glass plate, cover gel with cling film and cut gel strips 1.5 cm wide positioned 4–35 cm from origin with razor blade.

9. Transfer strips horizontally to clean glass plate (40 × 33 × 0.4 cm) 4 cm from edge. Put spacers (40 × 1 × 0.1 cm) on both edges vertically.

10. Put second glass plate on top. Seal plates with tape.

11. (a) Prepare second dimension gel (approximately 20 ml/gel) by mixing
    - 50 mM Tris–borate pH 8.3
    - 1 mM EDTA
    - 22.8% acrylamide
    - 0.8% *N,N'*-methylene bisacrylamide
    - 0.7 g/l APS
    (b) Filter through 0.45 μm nitrocellulose filter.
    (c) Start polymerization by adding TEMED (100 μl/l).

12. Pour gels up to 1 cm from top, filling all space around (and below) the

first dimension gel strip. Allow 30 min for polymerization. Remove tape from bottom.

13. Place gel plates in tank filled with running buffer (4–5 litres) consisting of
    - 50 ml Tris–borate pH 8.3
    - 1 mM EDTA

14. Connect through paper wick (Whatman 1MM) to upper reservoir (4).

15. Electrophorese at room temperature until bromophenol blue has moved 20–25 cm (run at 25 mA/gel for 5–7 h).

16. Remove one glass plate and cover gel with cling film. Autoradiograph at −70 °C for 1–4 days.

This method has been widely used to characterize the genomes of epidemiologically important viruses, like influenza viruses (11, 13–17) and poliomyelitis viruses (18, 19). Using oligonucleotide 'fingerprinting' and careful analysis of the autoradiographs it has been shown that influenza A viruses of subtypes H1N1 and H3N2 (14, 16) undergo constant evolution during circulation in the population. Surprisingly, it was found that oligonucleotide maps of H1N1 influenza A viruses which appeared in the winter of 1976–77 were genomically very closely related to H1N1 isolates obtained 26 years earlier during a period when these viruses were prevalent (1933–1956) (13). Since 1977 the subtypes of H1N1 and H3N2 of influenza A viruses have co-circulated. Oligonucleotide maps of isolated RNA segments were instrumental in detecting natural reassortant influenza viruses in 1978 which had part of their genome segments derived from H3N2 and part from H1N1 (15). Similarly, natural avian influenza virus isolates were found to be reassortants (11). Thus, molecular analysis of influenza A viruses has significantly contributed to knowledge of their epidemiology. Oligonucleotide maps of poliovirus genomes (18, 19) have helped to differentiate field strains and to recognize in the late 1970s that many isolates from cases of paralysis are more like the strains used for vaccination than like wild-type (18). Oligonucleotide maps of rotaviruses (20) also suggested reassortment *in vivo* long before this was confirmed by sequencing. Oligonucleotide mapping has also been used to differentiate retrovirus isolates (12, 21).

4. Analysis of restriction endonuclease fragments of DNA virus genomes by PAGE

The genomes of most animal DNA viruses are double-stranded and can therefore—after extraction—be cleaved by restriction endonucleases. The resulting fragments can be radiolabelled and analysed after separation by PAGE, and application of this procedure to clinical isolates has led to some important epidemiological findings. *Protocol 6* describes extraction of viral DNA, *Protocol 7* digestion with restriction endonucleases, and *Protocol 8* PAGE and autoradiography/staining.

Protocol 6. Extraction of viral DNA

A. *Herpesviruses* (reference 22)

1. Remove medium from herpes simplex virus (HSV)-infected cell cultures (BHK21 cells) (Linbro plates) showing approximately 50% cytopathic effect (CPE). (Viral DNA can be labelled by adding 50 μCi [^{32}P]orthophosphate (carrier-free, Amersham) 2–4 h after infection to phosphate-free medium.)

2. Transfer to Eppendorf tube, add 1 ml of phenol (saturated with 75 mM NaCl, 50 mM EDTA pH 8), mix, and keep on ice for 10 min.

3. Spin at 1500 *g* for 10 min.

4. Transfer aqueous phase into new tube, add 2 volumes of ethanol, mix, and spin at 1500 *g* for 10 min.

5. Discard supernatant; freeze-dry pellet.

6. Dissolve DNA pellet in 0.2 ml of distilled water containing 20 μg of RNase A (Sigma) and RNase T1 (200 units). Shake gently and incubate at 37 °C for 1–2 h.

B. *Adenoviruses* (reference 23)

1. Label adenovirus-infected cell cultures (293 cells) as under A1.

2. Extract low molecular weight DNA (reference 24): remove medium, and lyse cells in 0.4 ml of Tris–HCl buffer (10 mM, pH 7.4) containing 10 mM EDTA and 0.6% SDS for 10 min at room temperature.

3. Transfer lysate to an Eppendorf tube and add 0.1 ml of 5 M NaCl. Mix and keep at 4 °C overnight.

4. Remove high molecular weight cellular DNA by centrifugation at 11 000 *g* for 15 min in a microcentrifuge.

5. Digest supernatant with Proteinase K (Boehringer Mannheim, 500 μg/ml) for 3 h at 37 °C.

6. Extract twice with phenol:chloroform (1:1, v/v), and twice with ether.

7. Precipitate viral DNA with 2.5 volumes of ethanol. Mix and keep at −70 °C for 20 min. Pellet at 11 000 *g* for 15 min.

8. Vacuum dry pellet and dissolve in 50 ml of TE buffer (Tris–HCl buffer, 10 mM pH 7.4, 1 mM EDTA).

Protocol 7. Digestion of viral DNA with restriction endonucleases

1. Digest 5–10 μl aliquots of products of *Protocol 6* for 2–3 h with 2–4 units of restriction endonucleases in 50 μl volumes using buffers and conditions as indicated by the manufacturers. (In the case of material from *Protocol 6B*, add RNase A (Sigma, 20 μg per digest) after the RNase A stock has been boiled for 10 min.)

2. Add 5–10 μl (equal volume) of SBE running mixture consisting of 50% sucrose, 0.2% bromophenol blue, and 0.1 M EDTA pH 7.4.

3. Apply to horizontal 1–2% agarose gels (see *Protocol 8*).

Protocol 8. PAGE of DNA fragments and staining/ autoradiography

1. Dissolve 1.2–1.5 g of agarose (Sigma) in 100 ml of TBE buffer (10 mM Tris–borate pH 8, 1 mM EDTA). For DNA that is not radiolabelled, add 0.5 mg/ml of ethidium bromide. Boil for 5 min, then pour solution into minigel kit to achieve 3–5 mm thick gel. Allow to set.

2. Add sufficient TBE buffer to cover gel.

3. Add DNA fragments in SBE running mixture (5–10 μl) (see *Protocol 7*).

4. Apply voltage of 2 V/cm. Run at room temperature until bromophenol blue has reached bottom of gel.

5. If DNA is stained with ethidium bromide examine under UV light. When using ^{32}P-labelled DNA, transfer gel on to filter paper (Whatman no. 1), cover with cling film, dry in a vacuum gel drier (Bio-Rad), and auto-radiograph (−70 °C, intensifying screen).

PAGE of restriction endonuclease fragments has been used to analyse clinical isolates of HSV (22, 25), cytomegalovirus (CMV) (26, 27), and adenoviruses (23, 28). Thus it has been shown that restriction endonuclease fragment patterns of HSV-1 isolates show a great variability and are similar only for isolates obtained within close communities or clusters like families in which HSV very often seems to be passed on. In the rare cases of outbreaks caused by HSV, PAGE analysis of restriction fragments has been useful to analyse concomitant cases of encephalitis in hospital neonatal wards where more often than not it was found that cases were isolated incidents of infection and not epidemiologically connected (25). In cases of neonatal CMV infec-tions, close genomic relationship between the neonatal and the maternal isolates could be demonstrated (26), and chains of CMV infections could be followed in day-care centres (27). For adenoviruses, different 'genotypes' within different serotypes were demonstrated and periodical changes of different genotypes over time observed (23, 28).

5. Nucleic acid hybridization techniques

Techniques to produce complementary DNA (cDNA) from DNA or RNA templates, to radiolabel cDNA, and to use it as probe for hybridization have been described in detail in Chapter 3. Epidemiological applications have been particularly useful in situations where it has not been possible until now to grow viruses routinely in tissue culture (e.g. papillomaviruses, hepatitis B virus (HBV), and parvoviruses), where tissues expressing viral antigens are not easily available (HBV, parvoviruses, and some papillomaviruses) or where tissues are latently infected with viruses without expressing viral genes (papillomaviruses). The classification of papillomaviruses into over 60 human types (29) and correlation of infection with disease entities and epidemiological features (sexual transmission, family clusters, genetic susceptibility, geographic distribution, etc.) rested almost entirely on differentiation by cross-hybridization or the lack of it (30) and has only recently become more precise by applying the polymerase chain reaction (PCR) and sequencing techniques (29, 31).

6. Polymerase chain reaction

The PCR has been described in depth in Chapter 5. It is an extremely sensitive way of finding and amplifying a few viral genomes (or parts of it) within a vast excess of unrelated nucleic acid in extracts of infected tissue. Therefore—like hybridization techniques—it has been particularly useful in investigating infections with fastidious viruses (e.g. HBV, HPV, and parvoviruses) or viruses causing latent infections in their latent state (e.g. herpes viruses and some forms of measles). Reverse transcription (RT)-PCR, in which PCR is preceded by a RT step to produce cDNA from RNA templates, has, for example, been used to investigate infections with hepatitis C virus (HCV), which cannot be grown. The classification of HCV into at least six different types (32, 33) and the epidemiology (geographical distribution, transmission of certain types) are entirely based on the wide application of RT-PCR linked with partial sequencing (see below). The application of PCR and RT-PCR has also significantly contributed to the epidemiology of HIV infections. Using sets of *gag*-specific primers in PCRs on proviral DNA, seven distinct genotypes of HIV-1 have been differentiated so far (34) and aspects of their geographical distribution elucidated.

7. DNA sequencing

DNA sequencing is not a routine laboratory technique in the diagnostic laboratory, but as much of our knowledge on the molecular epidemiology of viruses has been obtained by sequence comparisons, some aspects of the technique will be dealt with here.

In many instances viral genes are cloned into plasmid vectors before sequencing. Description of cloning procedures is beyond the scope of this chapter, and reference is made to the comprehensive manual on molecular cloning by Sambrook *et al.* (2).

Amplification of viral genome sequences by PCR or RT-PCR yields enough material to set up DNA sequencing reactions directly (without the need for molecular cloning). This technique has come to be important in epidemiology and so will be briefly described. It involves firstly a DNA purification step and secondly a sequencing reaction; these are described in *Protocols 9* and *10*, respectively.

Protocol 9. Purification of DNA fragments obtained by PCR amplification

Principle

DNA is bound to a finely particulate slurry of glass powder in the presence of sodium iodide. Bound DNA is recovered by elution with distilled water.

Reagents ('Isogene' kit, Perkin-Elmer-Cetus)

- DNA binder slurry in water. Vortex immediately before use.
- Sodium iodide 6 M in 5 g/litre of a sodium sulphite solution. Keep in light tight bottle.

Keep all reagents at 2–8 °C.

- Wash buffer: Tris–HCl buffer 1 M, pH 7.5, containing 1 M NaCl and 100 mM EDTA. This is a 100 × concentrate to be diluted by a factor of 100 before use with 70% (v/v) ethanol.

Procedure

1. Place sample (20–500 µl) into 1.5 ml microcentrifuge tube. Add 2 volumes of 6 M sodium iodide. Cool to 4 °C (iced waterbath) for 5 min.

2. Add DNA binder (10 µl of slurry per 200 µl; for larger samples use 10 µl per 5 µl of DNA in sample). Mix gently for 10 min at room temperature to ensure binding of DNA.

3. Pellet bound DNA in microcentrifuge for 5 min. Remove supernatant carefully.

4. Wash pellet two or three times with 200 µl of wash buffer, resuspending the DNA binder slurry each time by vortexing for 5–10 sec followed by pelleting as in Step 3. (Resuspend and mix carefully to avoid possible shearing of long DNA molecules.)

183

Protocol 9. *Continued*

5. Remove supernatant from last wash. Release DNA by eluting in 20 µl of distilled water. Vortex and centrifuge as above. Collect supernatant and *repeat* elution step with another 20 µl of distilled water. (Typically, 10–15 % of bound DNA is eluted into the first 20 µl of water and 70–80 % into the second 20 µl of water.)

Note. The method can be modified to allow extraction of DNA bands from agarose gels followed by purification as shown above (Vogelstein and Gillespie (1979). *Proc. Natl. Acad. Sci. USA*, **76**, 615–19).

Protocol 10. Sequencing of purified DNA

1. Denature the DNA as described by Winship (35).
   (a) Pipette
      - DMSO, 1 µl
      - primer (25 ng), 1 µl
      - Sequenase buffer, 2 µl (10 mM Tris–HCl pH 7.5, 5 mM DTT, 0.5 mg/ml BSA)
      - PCR-amplified DNA 1–3 µl
      - water to 10 µl
   (b) Boil for 3 min and snap-cool in dry ice/ethanol bath.

2. Labelling/annealing reaction:
   (a) Add
      - 3 µl sequence enzyme/label mix (0.4 ml Sequenase (USB), 1 unit; 0.5 µl [^{35}S]dATP (5 µCi, sp. act. 1000 Ci/mM), and 2.1 µl of enzyme dilution buffer (see above))
      - 0.1 µl 0.l M of DTT
      - 2 µl of labelling mix consisting of 0.75 µM each of dGTP, dTTP, and dCTP (see reference 36)
      - 0.25 µl bacteriophage T7 gene 32 protein (Pharmacia) as described by Kaspar *et al.* (reference 37)
   (b) Mix and incubate for 3 min at room temperature.

3. Pipette one 3.5 µl aliquot (step 2) into each of four wells of a 96-well microtitre plate containing 2.5 µl Sequenase termination mix (80 µM dATP, dGTP, dCTP, dTTP plus 8 µM of one of the dideoxynucleotides ddATP, *or* ddGTP, *or* ddCTP, *or* ddTTP in 50 mM NaCl). Incubate at 37 °C for 10 min.

4. Add 7 µl of stop mix (90% formamide, 20 mM EDTA pH 8.0, 0.05% bromophenol blue, 0.05% xylene cyanol FF) to each well. Mix and

denature at 80 °C for 2 min. Cool on ice prior to loading (3 μl aliquots) to pre-run sequencing gels (see below).

5. (a) Prepare gel mix for sequencing gel (6% polyacrylamide), containing (per 500 ml)
   - acrylamide   28.5 g
   - *N,N′*-methylene bisacrylamide   1.5 g
   - urea   230 g
   - 5 × TBE   100 ml
   (1 × TBE: 90 mM Tris–borate pH 7.5, 2 mM EDTA)
   - Deionized water to 500 ml
   (b) Filter through Whatman no. 1 filter and store at 4 °C in the dark for up to 4 weeks.

6. Prepare gel plates using 0.37 mm wedge spacers and combs; tape edges and bottom.

7. For each ml of gel, add 2 μl of 25% APS and 2 μl of TEMED. Fill space between plates with gel (using a 50 ml syringe).

8. Pre-run gel using 1 × TBE buffer (see above) for 30 min.

9. Load samples (using a Hamilton syringe).

10. Run gel at 70 W constant until bromophenol blue reaches bottom.

11. Remove one plate, fix gel with acetic acid–ethanol–water (10:15:75), mount on Whatman 3MM paper, and cover with cling film. Dry under vacuum at 80 °C for 2 h.

12. Autoradiograph at − 70 °C using intensifying screen for 1–3 days (sometimes shorter).

Sequencing of parts of viral genomes has allowed various important conclusions to be drawn. For example comparisons of the haemagglutinin (HA) genes of influenza A virus H3N2 isolates obtained since 1968 has allowed the construction of evolutionary trees (see below) showing that the HA genes have changed over time in a directed way (38), confirming data obtained earlier for genome analysis of H1N1 viruses by oligonucleotide mapping (14). By contrast, influenza B and C viruses lack such directed evolution and showed co-circulation and co-evolution of viruses from different genetic origin (39).

Extensive sequence comparisons of parts of the HIV-1 genome have shown that wide differences are found not only for isolates from different geographical locations and times but also for sequential isolates from the same person; even within a single isolate, there can be virus particles of different genome composition. The 'quasispecies' character of HIV-1 isolates has been abundantly documented (40–48). Careful analyses of serial HIV specimens from

Table 1. Application of PCR to epidemiological surveillance of virus infections. (More recent applications continue to appear in the journals selected below)

Virus	Reference
CMV	Porter-Jordan, K. *et al.* (1990). *J. Med. Virol*, **30**, 85
Enteroviruses	Rotbart, H. A. (1990). *J. Clin. Microbiol.*, **28**, 438
	Chapman, N. M. *et al.* (1990). *J. Clin. Microbiol.*, **28**, 843
Flaviviruses	Eldalah, Z. A. *et al.* (1991). *J. Med. Virol.*, **33**, 260
HBV	Shih, L. N. *et al.* (1990). *J. Med. Virol.*, **30**, 159
	Norder, H. *et al.* (1990). *J. Med. Virol.*, **31**, 215
	Shih, L. N. *et al.* (1990). *J. Med. Virol.*, **32**, 257
HCV	Weiner, A. J. *et al.* (1990). *Lancet*, **I**, 1
	Garson, J. A. *et al.* (1990). *Lancet*, **I**, 1419
	Simmonds, P. *et al.* (1990). *Lancet*, **II**, 1469
HHV6	Kido, S. *et al.* (1990). *J. Med. Virol.*, **32**, 139
	Aubin, J. T. *et al.* (1991). *J. Clin. Microbiol.*, **29**, 367
HIV	Loche, M. and Mach, B. (1989). *Lancet*, **II**, 418
	Pezzella, M. *et al.* (1989). *Brit. Med. J.*, **298**, 713
	Rogers, M. F. *et al.* (1989). *N. Engl. J. Med.*, **320**, 1649
	Paterlini, P. *et al.* (1990). *J. Med. Virol.*, **30**, 53
	Sönnerborg, A. *et al.* (1990). *J. Med. Virol.*, **31**, 234
	Wages, J. M. *et al.* (1991). *J. Med. Virol.*, **33**, 58
	Dickover, R. E. *et al.* (1990). *J. Clin. Microbiol.*, **28**, 2130
	Albert, J. and Fenyö, E. M. (1990). *J. Clin. Microbiol.*, **28**, 1560
HPV	Young, L. S. *et al.* (1989). *Brit. Med. J.*, **298**, 14
	Syrjänen, S. *et al.* (1990). *J. Med. Virol.*, **31**, 259
	Morris, B. J. *et al.* (1990). *J. Med. Virol.*, **32**, 22
	Williamson, A. L. and Rubick, E. P. (1991). *J. Med. Virol.*, **33**, 165
HSV	Puchhamer-Stöckl, E. *et al.* (1990). *J. Med. Virol.*, **30**, 77
	Boermann, R. H. *et al.* (1991). *J. Med. Virol.*, **33**, 83
Measles (SSPE)	Godec, M. S. *et al.* (1990). *J. Med. Virol.*, **30**, 237
Parvovirus	Clewley, J. P. (1989). *J. Clin. Microbiol.*, **27**, 2647
	Koch, W. C. and Adler, S. P. (1990). *J. Clin. Microbiol.*, **28**, 65
Rotaviruses	Gouvea, V. *et al.* (1990). *J. Clin. Microbiol.*, **28**, 276
VZV	Kido, S. *et al.* (1991). *J. Clin. Microbiol.*, **29**, 76

individual patients have also led to the conclusion that divergent and convergent evolution happen side by side simultaneously (49). These findings have important implications for the epidemiology of HIV infections: when the virus is transmitted the development of infection and disease may depend on which mutants are transmitted and how they evolve in the new host. The quasispecies character of HIV may in part explain the very wide variance of incubation periods and outcome of infection in terms of symptomatology. It makes the allocation of epidemiological and pathological characteristics to certain mutants a daunting task (see below).

From comparative sequence information, specific primers can be designed for PCR, which will yield type-specific products. Thus, without sequencing, a certain degree of genotyping is possible by screening isolates obtained in epidemiological contexts; the method has been used for HIV (34), HCV (32), rotaviruses (50), and a variety of other viruses. Examples are given in *Table 1*. If the primers for PCR are chosen to amplify parts of the genome coding for serotype-specifying epitopes, genotyping by PCR can be correlated well with serotypes (50) and in part replace serological procedures.

8. Monoclonal antibodies

Monoclonal antibodies (mAbs) (51) are used in serological procedures (see Chapter 1), but as the epitopes they react with can be defined in molecular terms in many cases or at least be determined as confirmational sites, use of mAbs in epidemiological contexts can be regarded as part of molecular epidemiology. The production and analysis of mAbs has been the object of various monographs (e.g. 52) and the reader is referred to them for more detailed information.

MAbs have been widely used to characterize viral isolates obtained from outbreaks and to compare them. For influenza viruses it has been shown that the antigenic sites of neutralizing mAbs detected by sequence analysis of the HA genes of *in vitro* 'escape' mutants and the antigenic sites which changed during circulation within an HA subtype were identical (53) suggesting that for influenza A viruses selection by circulating antibody played a role in the evolution of these viruses.

Panels of neutralizing mAbs (which constantly increase) are being used to serotype certain viruses like rotaviruses (54) using neutralization tests (Chapter 1) or ELISAs (Chapter 2). These procedures allow the study of the geographical distribution of rotaviruses and have indicated the co-circulation of serotypes with prevalences in unpredictable ratios all over the world (54). Such data are of great importance when developing a strategy for vaccines (55).

The sequences of wild-type polioviruses and the live attenuated vaccine counterparts have been determined for all three types. If poliovirus-associated paralytic disease is diagnosed in a widely vaccinated population it is crucial to establish quickly whether the poliovirus isolates of clinical cases are associated with the vaccine or the wild-type. The use of panels of mAbs raised against vaccine and wild-type viruses allows a quick decision to be made in this respect (56).

9. Virus evolution

Viruses, particularly RNA viruses, evolve rapidly, and a thorough under-standing of the mechanisms underlying these changes is important not only from the point of view of basic knowledge but also for the planning of preventive measures. Details of methodological aspects of this analysis are given in chapter 8.

10. Molecular pathology

Molecular data on viruses are increasingly being used in order to explore mechanisms of viral spread and development of disease. Many aspects of this are dealt with in ref. 57. Examples of this approach are:

(a) The use of monoreassortants to elucidate the pathogenesis of central nervous system infections with reoviruses in mice (58) or of infections with rotaviruses in animals (59, 60).

(b) Analysis of the *env* genes of HIV isolates from brain and other tissues to locate organotropic sequences (46).

(c) Analysis of the *M* genes of measles virus obtained from acute infections and from SSPE cases (61).

References

1. Lustig, A. and Levine, A. J. (1992). *J. Virol.*, **66**, 4629.
2. Sambrook, J., Fritsch, E. F., and Maniatis, T. (1989). *Molecular cloning. A laboratory manual*. 2nd edn. Cold Spring Harbor Laboratory Press, Cold Spring Harbor, NY.
3. Whitton, J. L., Hundley, F., O'Donnell, B., and Desselberger, U. (1983). *J. Virol. Methods*, **7**, 183.
4. Espejo, R. T., Muñoz, O., Serafin, F., and Romero, P. (1980). *Infect. Immun.*, **27**, 351.
5. Rodger, S. M., Bishop, R. F., Birch, L., McLean, B., and Holmes, I. H. (1981). *J. Clin. Microbiol.*, **13**, 272.
6. Follett, E. A. C., Sanders, R. C., Beards, G. M., Hundley, F., and Desselberger, U. (1984). *J. Hyg. (Camb.)*, **92**, 209.
7. Desselberger, U. (1989). In *Viruses and the gut* (ed. M. J. G. Farthing), pp. 55–65. Swan Press, London.
8. Beards, G. M., Desselberger, U., and Flewett, T. H. (1989). *J. Clin. Microbiol.*, **27**, 2827.
9. Beards, G. M. (1982). *Arch. Virol.*, **74**, 65.
10. Pedley, S., Hundley, F., Chrystie, I., McCrae, M. A., and Desselberger, U. (1984). *J. Gen. Virol.*, **65**, 1141.
11. Desselberger, U., Nakajima, K., Alfino, P., Pedersen, F. S., Haseltine, W. A., Hannoun, C., and Palese, P. (1978). *Proc. Natl. Acad. Sci. USA*, **75**, 3341.
12. Pedersen, F. S. and Haseltine, W. A. (1980). In *Methods in enzymology* (ed. L. Grossman and K. Moldave), Vol. 65, pp. 680–7. Academic Press, New York.
13. Nakajima, K., Desselberger, U., and Palese, P. (1978). *Nature*, **274**, 334.
14. Young, J. F., Desselberger, U., and Palese, P. (1979). *Cell*, **18**, 73.
15. Young, J. F. and Palese, P. (1979). *Proc. Natl. Acad. Sci. USA*, **76**, 6547.

16. Ortin, J., Najera, R., Lopez, C., Davila, M., and Domingo, E. (1980). *Gene*, **11**, 319.
17. Guo, Y. J. and Desselberger, U. (1984). *J. Gen. Virol.*, **65**, 1857.
18. Nottay, B. K., Kew, O. M., Hatch, M. H., Heyward, J. T., and Obijeski, J. F. (1981). *Virology*, **108**, 405.
19. Minor, P. D. (1982). *J. Gen. Virol.*, **59**, 307.
20. Desselberger, U., Hung, T., and Follet, E. A. C. (1986). *Virus Res.*, **4**, 357.
21. Chen, E., Peters, W. P., Sweet, R. W., Ohno, T., Kufe, D. W., Spiegelman, S., *et al.* (1976). *Nature*, **260**, 266.
22. Lonsdale, D. M. (1979). *Lancet*, **i**, 849.
23. O'Donnell, B., Bell, E., Payne, S. B., Mautner, V., and Desselberger, U. (1986). *J. Med. Virol.*, **18**, 213.
24. Hirt, B. (1967). *J. Mol. Biol.*, **26**, 365.
25. Roizman, B. and Buchman, T. (1979). *Hospital Practice*, **14**, 95.
26. Huang, E., Alford, C. A., Reynolds, D. W., Stagno, S., and Pass, R. F. (1980). *N. Engl. J. Med.*, **303**, 958.
27. Adler, S. P. (1991). *Pediatr. Infect. Dis. J.*, **10**, 584.
28. Wadell, G. (1984). *Curr. Top. Microbiol. Immunol.*, **110**, 140.
29. Chan, S. Y., Bernard, H. U., Ong, C. K., Chan, S. P., Hofmann, B., and Delius, H. (1992). *J. Virol.*, **66**, 5714.
30. de Villiers, E. M. (1989). *J. Virol.*, **63**, 4898.
31. Schiffman, M. H., Bauer, H. M., Lorincz, A. T., Manos, M. M., Byrne, J. C., Glass, A. G., *et al.* (1991). *J. Clin. Microbiol.*, **29**, 573.
32. Simmonds, P., McOmish, F., Yap. P. L., Chan, S. W., Lin, C. K., Dusheiko, G., *et al.* (1993). *J. Gen. Virol.*, **74**, 661.
33. Okamoto, H., Kojima, M., Sakamoto, M., Iizula, H., Hadiwandowo, S., Suwignyo, S., *et al.* (1994). *J. Gen. Virol.*, **75**, 629.
34. Louwagie, J., McCutchan, F. E., Peeters, M., Brennan, T. P., Sanders-Buell, E., Eddy, G. A., *et al.* (1993). *AIDS*, **7**, 769.
35. Winship, P. R. (1989). *Nucleic Acids Res.*, **17**, 1266.
36. Tsang, T. C. and Bentley, D. R. (1988). *Nucleic Acids Res.*, **16**, 6238.
37. Kasper, P., Zadvil, S., and Febry, M. (1989). *Nucleic Acids Res.*, **17**, 3616.
38. Both, G. W., Sleigh, M. J., Cox, N. J., and Kendal, A. P. (1983). *J. Virol.*, **48**, 52.
39. Yamashita, M., Krystal, M., Fitch, W. M., and Palese, P. (1988). *Virology*, **163**, 112.
40. Hahn, B. H., Shaw, G. M., Taylor, M. E., Redfield, R. L., Markham, P. D., Salahuddin, S. Z., *et al.* (1986). *Science*, **232**, 1548.
41. Koyanagi, Y., Miles, S., Mitsuyasa, R. T., Merril, J. E., Winters, J. V., and Chen, S. Y. (1987). *Science*, **286**, 819.
42. Chiodi, F., Valentin, A., Keys, B., Schwartz, S., Asjö, B., Gartner, S., *et al.* (1988). *Virology*, **173**, 178.
43. La Rosa, G. J., Davide, J. P., Weinhold, K., Waterbury, J. A., Profy, A. T., Lewis, J. A., *et al.* (1990). *Science*, **249**, 932.
44. Simmonds, P., Balfe, P., Ludlam, C. A., Bishop, J. O., and Leigh Brown, A. J. (1990). *J. Virol.*, **64**, 5840.
45. Meyerhans, A., Cheynier, R., Albert, J., Seth, M., Kwok, S., Sninsky, J., *et al.* (1989). *Cell*, **58**, 901.
46. Epstein, L. G., Kuitken, C., Blumberg, B. M., Hartman, S., Sharer, L. R., Clement, M., and Goutsmit, J. (1991). *Virology*, **180**, 583.

47. Martins, L. J., Chenciner, N., Asjö, B., Meyerhans, A., and Wain-Hobson, S. (1991). *J. Virol.*, **65**, 4502.

48. Wolfs, F. W., de Jong, J. J., van den Berg, H., Tijnagel, J. M. G. H., Krone, W. J. A., and Goutsmit, J. (1990). *Proc. Natl. Acad. Sci. USA*, **87**, 9938.

49. Holmes, E. C., Zhang, L. Q., Simmonds, P., Ludlam, C. A., and Leigh Brown, A. J. (1992). *Proc. Natl. Acad. Sci. USA*, **89**, 4835.

50. Gouvea, V. S., Glass, R. I., Woods, P., Taniguchi, K., Clark, H. F., Forrester, B., and Fang, Z. Y. (1990). *J. Clin. Microbiol.*, **28**, 276.

51. Köhler, G. and Milstein, C. (1975). *Nature*, **256**, 495.

52. Goding, J. W. (1986). *Monoclonal antibodies: principles and practice*. Academic Press, London.

53. Webster, R. G., Lever, W. G., and Air, G. M. (1983). In *Genetics of Influenza Viruses* (ed. P. Palese and W. Kingsbury), pp. 127–68. Springer-Verlag, Wien and New York.

54. Kapikian, A. Z. and Chanock, R. M. (1990). In *Virology* (ed. B. N. Fields, D. M. Knight, R. M. Chanock, M. S. Hirsch, J. L. Melnick, T. P. Monath, and B. Roizman), pp. 1353–404. Raven Press, New York.

55. Desselberger, U. (1993). *Reviews Med. Virol.*, **3**, 15.

56. Ferguson, M. (1990). Pers. Communication.

57. Oldstone, M. B. A. (ed.) (1990). *Animal virus pathogenesis: A practical approach*. IRL Press, Oxford.

58. Sharpe, A. H. and Fields, B. N. (1985). *N. Engl. J. Med.*, **312**, 486.

59. Offit, P. A., Blavat, G., Greenberg, H. B., and Clark, H. F. (1986). *J. Virol.*, **57**, 46.

60. Bridger, J., Burke, B., Beards, G., and Desselberger, U. (1992). *J. Gen. Virol.*, **73**, 3011–15.

61. Cattaneo, R., Schmid, A., Eschle, D., Baczko, K., ter Meulen, V., and Billeter, M. A. (1988). *Cell*, **55**, 255.

8

Evolutionary analysis of viruses

ANDREW J. LEIGH BROWN

1. Introduction

There are many reasons why a clear understanding of the genetic relationship between different strains of a virus and of their evolution is desirable. It can provide information on the origins and geographical distribution of particular strains, on routes of transmission, and for the development of vaccines. With the increasingly widespread use of rapid nucleotide sequencing methods, and particularly since the advent of the polymerase chain reaction, extensive genetic data have been obtained on many viruses. Whereas previously mainly serological methods may have been used to distinguish strains, detecting limited numbers of variable epitopes, a much more complete description of the relatedness between strains using genetic analysis is now possible. This has been particularly prominent in the analysis of the evolution and origins of influenza viruses (1–7) and of human immunodeficiency virus type 1 (HIV-1), where the determination of relatedness by sequence analysis has preceded a successful serological classification (8–14). Recently there have been signifi- cant developments in the phylogenetic analysis of other viruses as well, notably papillomaviruses, feline immunodeficiency virus, and hepatitis C virus (15–17).

The principles involved in the analysis of genetic relationships between viral strains, or phylogenies, are similar whether the data consist of oligo- nucleotide fragments, restriction endonuclease fragments, or nucleotide sequences. Evolution is conventionally described in terms of a bifurcating tree. While not necessarily formally correct in all cases (as strong selection can cause significant deviation from a continuously divergent tree), it will be assumed for the purposes of this discussion. However, in all phylogenetic comparisons it is necessary to be confident that the sequences being compared between strains did at some point derive from a common ancestral gene, i.e. that they are truly *homologous*. By virtue of this definition, homology is an all-or-none state, therefore the phrase 'percent homology' is an oxymoron. It is more appropriate to refer to 'percent identity'. If amino acids are grouped on the basis of physico-chemical characteristics, 'percent similarity' can be used to refer to more distantly related proteins.

Phylogenetic trees can be either rooted, which implies that the direction of evolution is known *a priori*, or unrooted, when it is not. In practice it is often most appropriate to adopt a procedure which gives an unrooted tree but to impose a root by including an 'outgroup'—perhaps a strain that is clearly the most distant relative of those whose relationships are under investigation. The major practical problems associated with the inference of phylogenies are:

(a) the number of possible trees from which the correct tree has to be chosen

(b) branching not diverging continually, often because strains vary in their rate of change

(c) incomplete sampling of the tree

The last is an issue in data collection but the first two are problems of analysis and will be discussed in more detail.

1.1. The number of evolutionary trees

It is often not fully appreciated how many possible trees exist which could describe the relationships between even small numbers of strains. The number of unrooted trees is given by: $\Pi(2i-1)$ where i takes values from 1 to $n-2$ (Π is the symbol for multiplication, as Σ is the symbol for summation; n is the number of strains). In *Table 1* these figures are given for 3–10 strains (18). The number of possible unrooted trees for n strains is the same as the number of rooted trees for $n-1$ strains. For 20 strains the number of possible different unrooted trees will be approximately 3×10^{23}. With rapid sequencing methods becoming widely used, data sets containing sequences of substantially more than 20 strains are being generated. Clearly, any complete evaluation of that number of topologies is impossible, and in general terms strategies must be used which can find the 'correct' tree by searching only a subset of all possible trees.

Table 1. Number of unrooted trees for 3–10 strains

Number of strains (n)	Number of unrooted trees
3	1
4	3
5	15
6	105
7	945
8	10 395
9	1.4×10^5
10	2.0×10^6

1.2 Divergent and convergent evolution

In the simplest evolutionary models, it is assumed that all changes are unique and that no reversion or back-mutation occurs at any site in the entire phylogeny. The branches of the tree will therefore continually diverge from each other and all data sets obtained from the genomes being studied (for example from different genes) will give the same topology. This view is completely appropriate only when individual characters are so complex that they are only likely to arise once. For molecular data, where characters are nucleotides, amino acids, or restriction sites, this is not the case. For example, a particular restriction site could be lost in parallel on different branches of the tree, but is less likely to be reacquired. With sequence data, and especially for nucleotide sequences, it is quite likely that a given site could undergo parallel changes in different branches or take different paths before reaching the same state (convergence). Three different approaches to phylogenetic analysis have been developed which attempt, in different ways, to deal with the very large number of possible trees and the problem of convergence. These are discussed in the following sections.

2. Measures of genetic distance

One set of methods has been developed based on estimates of the pairwise genetic similarity (or distance) between strains. These originated in work on the classification of bacteria (19), but more recently metrics of similarity for restriction site (20) and nucleotide and amino acid sequence data (21, 22) have been developed. Calculation of the metric for all pairwise comparisons of strains reduces the data to a single figure for each comparison. This generates a 'distance matrix' which then forms the basis for estimation of the evolutionary relationships.

2.1 Estimation of nucleotide distance

To an increasing extent the data becoming available for analysis of relationships between virus strains consist of nucleotide sequences. While they certainly provide the most complete and direct information about genetic relationships, nucleotide sequences suffer from an important limitation at the analysis stage. Because of the small number of possible character states—the four nucleotides—evolutionary convergence onto the same state by two unrelated sequences will occur relatively frequently. This will result in a significant *underestimation* of genetic distances, a bias which will increase when distantly related strains, or rapidly evolving genes, are being considered. It is not sufficient, therefore, simply to adopt a measure based on the observed similarity between strains; rather it is essential to estimate the real divergence from the data using one of several estimators which make some form of correction for 'multiple hits', i.e. multiple substitutions at the same residue (see the recent review by Gojobori *et al.* (reference 23)). Those in most common use are the 'one-parameter' model of Jukes and Cantor (18) and the 'two-parameter' model of Kimura (19). In the former it is assumed that any nucleotide is equally likely to be substituted by any other. In this case the estimated number of nucleotide substitutions (K) which have occurred since two strains diverged is given by:

$$K = -3/4 \ln(1 - 4/3\lambda) \qquad [1]$$

where λ is the observed fraction of sites at which the two sequences differ.

In the two-parameter model, transitions (purine–purine and pyrimidine–pyrimidine substitutions) and transversions (purine–pyrimidine and pyrimidine–purine substitutions) are considered separately. The estimate of the mean number of nucleotide substitutions is then:

$$K = 1/2 \ln[(1 - 2P - Q) \sqrt{(1 - 2Q)}] \qquad [2]$$

where P is the fraction of sites at which the two sequences differ by a transition substitution and Q is the fraction at which they differ by a transversion; $P + Q = \lambda$. When transitions and transversions differ in frequency then an improvement in the estimate can be obtained by using the Kimura expression (19).

However sophisticated the estimator, there are biologically realistic situations where no correction will work well: when the probability of substitution varies according to position, all will give an underestimate because they average across the entire sequence. This effect can be quite serious. For example, in the case of the V4-C3-V5 regions of the *env* gene of HIV-1 analysed by Balfe *et al.* (12) where two rapidly evolving regions flank a conserved sequence, it would be appropriate to subdivide the sequence for analysis into rapidly and slowly evolving segments.

In protein-coding sequences where the amino acid sequence is relatively conserved, synonymous substitutions (those nucleotide substitutions which do not change an amino acid) and non-synonymous substitutions (those which lead to an amino acid change) should be considered separately (9, 24). Synonymous substitutions are then usually used in the estimation of evolutionary distance, because they are less affected by variation in the rate of change. A good example is the investigation of sequence variability in Newcastle disease virus by Sakaguchi *et al.* (25).

2.2 Phylogenies from distance matrices

Once a distance matrix has been constructed the phylogeny can be inferred by applying one of a variety of clustering procedures. Several simple cluster analysis methods are available which give a representation of these relationships.

One of the simplest is the UPGM (unweighted pair-group mean) method (16). Developed to represent the phenotypic distance between organisms, this often-used method is limited in its value in evolutionary analyses, as it assumes equal rates of change down different branches of the phylogenetic tree.

The method begins with a distance matrix such as that shown below:

Strain	A	B	C
B	4		
C	9	7	
D	20	18	17

From such a matrix, the two strains with the smallest distance (d) are grouped. In this case, strains A and B are grouped together: as the rate of evolution is assumed to be constant, the branch length to each from their common ancestor, $d_{AB}/2$, is 2 units. A new matrix is now constructed treating A and B as a single composite group. The distances from the composite group (AB) to the other strains is taken as the arithmetic mean of their individual distances from A and B, i.e.:

$$d_{(AB)C} = (d_{AC} + d_{AB})/2$$

In this case the new matrix is therefore:

Strain	(AB)	C
C	8	
D	19	17

Again, the two closest units, (AB) and C, are grouped. The distance from each to their common ancestor is determined: $(d_{AC} + d_{BC})/2 \times 1/2 = 4$. The mean distance of the new composite group [(AB)C] to D, $(d_{(AB)D} + d_{CD})/2 = 18$ and so the branch length to D is 9 units. By convention, the tree is rooted at the midpoint of the longest branch. The tree therefore looks like that shown in *Figure 1*.

When the UPGM method is used, a substantial amount of information can

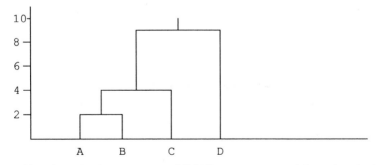

Figure 1. Unweighted pair-group mean (UPGM) tree constructed from data in the distance matrix in Section 2.2.

be lost if rates of change differ between branches. This can readily be demonstrated by clustering the same strains using the method devised by Fitch and Margoliash (26) which allows rates of change to differ within the tree, rather than assuming them to be equal. According to this method we estimate the branch lengths *a* and *b* leading to strains A and B from their common ancestor (node) α and we use the distances from each of A and B to C to do this, which correspond to $(a + x)$ and $(b + x)$ as shown below:

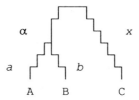

The leg lengths are estimated from a simple series of simultaneous equations as follows:

$$a + b = 4$$
$$a + x = 9$$
$$b + x = 7$$

These equations are solved to:

$$a - b = 2$$

so $a = 3$, $b = 1$, and $x = 6$.

Thus, the branch lengths *a* and *b* are not equal. The method proceeds as before by grouping A and B together and rewriting the matrix using the mean of their distances to the other groups. The second matrix is therefore identical to that given for the UPGM method. Again simultaneous equations permit the estimation of the branch length, *d*, from C to the common ancestor, β, and of C and the branches leading to A and B:

$$c + d = 8$$
$$c + e = 19$$
$$d + e = 17$$

196

These equations are solved to:

$$c - d = 2$$

so $c = 5$, $d = 3$, and $e = 14$.

We can now place the two nodes, α and β, on the tree as the distance between them is given by $x - d = 3$.

Combining the trees we obtain a tree as shown in *Figure 2*.

Even using this simple data set the tree is rather different from that given in *Figure 1*. While this procedure is clearly better, it still assumes additivity in the data, and substantial departures from this will result in negative branch lengths.

A more recent procedure which is extremely fast and highly efficient at finding the correct tree is the neighbour-joining method (27), which sequentially finds the nearest pairs of neighbouring sequences which give the shortest overall length of the tree. For a comparison of these methods and an excellent introduction to molecular phylogenetics, the reader is referred to Li and Graur (28). A more detailed review of phylogenetic methods suitable for molecular data can be found in reference 29.

3. Character-based methods

3.1 Maximum parsimony trees

The most popular approach to phylogeny reconstruction currently in use is that based on the principle of 'maximum parsimony'. Unlike distance methods, parsimony methods are 'character-based' and examine each site (character) in a sequence separately. Under the parsimony principle it is assumed that the 'best' tree is that which has the shortest *overall* length; the aim, therefore, is to minimize the number of convergent substitutions. The principle behind the parsimony approach is as follows (18): the data are reduced first by elimination of all invariant sites and second by removal of those where the variant residues (nucleotides or amino acids) are found only

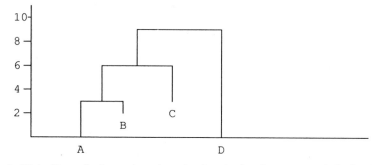

Figure 2. Fitch–Margoliash tree based on the data in the distance matrix in Section 2.2.

Table 2.

Strain	Sequence
a	T A C T C G G
b	T T A C A C G
c	G T A C A C G
d	G A A C T C G
Site:	1 2 3 4 5 6 7

in a single sequence. Sites where two or more residues are each represented more than once in the data, are termed 'phylogenetically informative'. The tree topology which minimizes the total number of substitutions at these sites is selected. Quite often it is found that there is not one single most parsimonious tree, in which case some additional criteria might be used to distinguish the alternatives. In *Table 2* four seven-nucleotide sequences are shown of which site 7 has no variation, and sites 3, 4, and 6 only distinguish a single sequence. Three sites (1, 2, and 5) are phylogenetically informative. At these three sites strains b and c shared nucleotides at both positions 2 and 5, while strains (a and b) and (c and d) share nucleotides at position 1 only. The tree with the smallest number of changes overall is then adopted. In this simple case the parsimony tree takes a linear structure shown in *Figure 3*.

The number of changes in each branch between a pair can be deduced by comparison of the sequences involved together with those of the nearest neighbour. Thus, b and c are grouped together, but to determine on which branch from node α the T/G change at site 1 occurred they are compared with sequence d. As this has a G at this site, this is deduced to be the ancestral state and the change is assigned to branch b, written as '1,1', indicating one change at site 1, with the ancestral sequence being GTACACG. Using sequence a in the same way allows the common ancestral sequence at node β to be partly reconstructed. At site 2, sequences b and c both have T, while

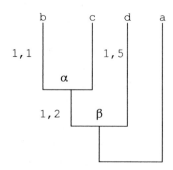

Figure 3. Maximum parsimony tree based on the data in the distance matrix in Table 2.

sequence d has an A. As sequence a also has A this is deduced to be the ancestral state, and the change at this site is assigned to the internode between β and α. However, no decision can be reached on these data regarding site 5 so the ancestral sequence at β is written GAACA/TCG.

In data sets where evolution is generally divergent in pattern, parsimony methods may perform well and not only give a good estimate of the correct tree but also of the branch lengths. Under such circumstances the programs in the PAUP package distributed by David Swofford (see Section 6.2 for details) will be particularly useful because of their speed of execution and ease of use, and their use was demonstrated in the analysis of sequence diversity in Type 3 reoviruses (30).

3.2 Limitations to parsimony

The circumstances where parsimony methods will not perform well are those in which there are large numbers of convergent substitutions in the data. This is particularly relevant when evolution is rapid and variable in rate (31). In influenza A viruses and HIV-1, regions of certain proteins where rapid change is observed have been implicated as being involved in escape from immune selection (1, 32, 33). If there are also constraints on the direction of sequence change, convergent substitution will occur. Parsimony methods are then likely to give the wrong tree because they are intended to minimize the number of such events. Recent results obtained for the V3 hypervariable region of gp120 in HIV-1 suggest that such effects do occur (14).

4. Statistical significance of tree topologies

4.1 Bootstrapping

The topology obtained by any of these procedures should be viewed only as an estimate of the phylogenetic relationships between a group of strains or sequences. In the interpretation of the tree it is important to know whether two groups on the tree are really distinct, or whether their apparent separation falls within the error associated with estimating the tree. Most methods for estimating tree topologies do not give any information on the statistical significance of their structure. This limitation has usually been dealt with by the use of a non-parametric statistical procedure known as bootstrapping to evaluate the significance of a particular topology (34).

Bootstrapping involves resampling the data on which the tree was based to generate a distribution of data sets from each of which a new tree is determined. The frequency with which particular branches are observed in the resampled data sets then allow probability statements to be attached to them in the original tree. This procedure is highly suitable for use in conjunction with parsimony and neighbour-joining procedures and should be incorporated into all studies based on them as a matter of routine.

4.2 Maximum likelihood trees

An alternative approach to phylogenetic inference based on maximum likelihood estimation has the very important advantage in that it immediately provides an estimate of the probability associated with a given branch or internode distance. In addition, it can be used to evaluate the relative likelihoods of two different topologies.

Maximum likelihood procedures involve the estimation of the likelihood of particular tree given a certain model of nucleotide substitution (35, 36). Their advantages are threefold. First, they are based on an explicit model of sequence evolution, which can in principle be tailored to the particular problem under investigation. Secondly, likelihood procedures associate a probability statement with each internodal segment, as indicated above. Thirdly, in contrast to distance matrix methods, the complete nucleotide sequence information is used in the determination of the phylogeny. However, the individual computations of likelihood are very time-consuming and the use of the likelihood approach has generally been restricted to small data sets. With the increasing availability of fast workstations such as the SUN SPARC station which can be dedicated to such problems, the DNAML likelihood program in the PHYLIP 3.5 package (see below) should become applicable to much larger data sets.

4.3 Conclusion

Any tree, whether it is 'most parsimonious' or has the 'maximum likelihood', is no more than a working hypothesis as to the relationships between a set of strains or species. All methods make some assumptions about the nature of the evolutionary process. Therefore, in order to increase confidence in the result, it is advisable to use more than one for all major analyses. Concordance between different methods will add significantly to one's confidence in the result, while differences may point up some interesting features of the data, such as convergence arising from selection.

5. Software for phylogenetic analyses

There is a large choice of methods available for phylogenetic analyses, many of which incorporate the parsimony principle. Programs for executing such methods, which can often be run within a reasonable time on a personal computer, can be selected from software packages distributed at little if any cost by Drs Joe Felsenstein ('PHYLIP' (PHYLogenetic Inference Package), version 3.4), and D. Swofford ('PAUP' (phylogenetic analysis using parsimony), version 3.0) at the addresses given below. Other programs which might be considered include 'MacClade', written for Apple Macintosh computers by Wayne Maddison at the University of Arizona (suitable for character-state data only); 'CLUSTAL' (reference 37), a multiple alignment program developed by Dr Desmond Higgins, now at EMBL, which estimates phylogenies while aligning sequences and now incorporates the neighbour-joining procedure with a bootstrap analysis; and 'TreeAlign', which is similar to CLUSTAL, was developed by Dr Jotun Hein and is also now available from EMBL. It should be noted that confidence intervals cannot be placed on the phylogenies produced by simultaneous alignment/tree-building programs.

5.1 PHYLIP 3.5

This is a comprehensive and well-supported package of tree-building programs based on a wide variety of approaches including distance matrix (e.g. Fitch–Margoliash and neighbour-joining) and maximum likelihood methods as well as parsimony. It is well-documented and easier to use than previous releases. Version 3.5 is written in C and Pascal and is available at no charge from Dr Joe Felsenstein, Department of Genetics SK-50, University of Washington Seattle, Wa 98195, USA (e-mail (EARN/BITNET): FELSENST@UWAVM or: joe%genetics.washington.edu@CUNYVM.CUNY.EDU). There are also executable versions available, or becoming available, for PC DOS and Apple Macintosh systems. PHYLIP 3.5 can be most efficiently obtained in compressed format by anonymous FTP from evolution.genetics.washington.edu (code 128.95.12.41).

Having made sure that sufficient memory is available (about 5 Mb), proceed as in *Protocol 1*.

Protocol 1. Using PHYLIP 3.5

1. Type 'Anonymous' in response to the **Login** prompt and your last name in response to the **password** prompt.

2. Type 'cd pub' to enter the directory 'pub'.

3. Prepare FTP for transfer of binary data

4. Tell FTP to get the following files:
   (a) working from UNIX systems:
   - 'phylip.tar.Z' (source code and documentation) and
   - 'phylipxp.tar.Z' (PC DOS executable object files)
   (b) working from PC DOS systems:
   - 'phylip.arc' (source code and documentation) and
   - 'phylipxp.arc (PC DOS executable object files)
   (These are self-extracting 'Zoo' files)
   (c) 'phylip.readme' contains detailed instructions (of which these are a brief summary)

5. Leave FTP.

Protocol 1. *Continued*

6. On a UNIX system use the 'uncompress' facility to generate the individual files. On a PC DOS system the Zoo archive file will self-extract when executed in its own directory as if it were a program. At the time of writing, PHYLIP version 3.5 is about to be released.

5.2 PAUP

This is a highly developed parsimony program of great flexibility which can find out most parsimonious trees and estimate confidence intervals by bootstrapping. It is much faster than the parsimony programs in PHYLIP. Available for US$50 from: Dr D. Swofford, Center for Biodiversity, Natural Resources Building, 607 East Peabody Drive, Champaign, Illinois 61820, USA. PAUP Version 3 is now available for Apple Macintosh computers. At present only version 2 is available for PC DOS but apparently a PC DOS version 3.0 will also soon be released.

5.3 MacClade

This was written by Wayne Maddison and David Maddison of the University of Arizona. All distribution is by Sinauer Associates, Sunderland, Massachusetts 01375, USA, Tel. (413) 665 3722; Fax (413) 665 7292. MacClade enables the use of the mouse–window interface to specify and rearrange phylogenies by hand, and to watch the number of character steps and the distribution of states of a given character on the tree change.

5.4. Hennig86

This is a fast parsimony program produced by J. S. Farris. It is distributed by Arnold Kluge, Amphibians and Reptiles, Museum of Zoology, University of Michigan, Ann Arbor, Michigan 48109-1079, USA. It runs on PCs under DOS.

5.5 CLUSTAL and TreeAlign

TreeAlign is available from the EMBL net server: e-mail (EARN/BITNET): 'NETSERV@EMBL'. Under 'subject' in the e-mail message enter 'help software'. CLUSTAL is available from Dr Desmond Higgins (e-mail (EARN/BITNET): higgins@EMBL) and also by anonymous FTP at the Indiana, Houston, and EMBL molecular biology distribution sites. Their network addresses are respectively: ftp.bio.indiana.edu, ftp.bchs.uh.edu, and ftp.embl-heidelberg.de. In the Indiana archive one must enter directory molbio/align, in the Houston archive it is in directory pub/gene-server in all of the four directories dos, Mac, unix, and vms, and on the EMBL archive it is in pub/software/unix or pub/software/vax.

5.6 Molecular evolutionary genetic analysis (MEGA)

This will analyse data from DNA, RNA, and protein sequences, and distance matrices produced from other kinds of data as well. It will include the neighbour-joining method, distance matrix method, a branch and bound parsimony method, and bootstrapping. It will run on PC DOS and will also plot trees on many kinds of printers. It was released at the beginning of 1993 by Sudhir Kumar, Koichiro Tamura, and Masatoshi Nei of the Institute of Molecular Evolutionary Genetics, 328 Mueller Laboratory, Pennsylvania State University, University Park, Pennsylvania 16802, USA. It is being provided free of charge if you send one 1.2 Mb 5.25 inch or 1.44 Mb 3.5 inch floppy diskette to M. Nei at the above address or contact him by electronic mail at nxm2@psuvm (Bitnet) or nxm2@psuvm.psu.edu (Internet).

5.7 Genetic data environment (GDE)

This is produced by Steve Smith, formerly of the Harvard Genome Laboratory. This is an interactive sequence editor for X-windows (SUN) which allows the user to edit sequences and align them by hand, and to select subsets of sites and sequences and call a variety of analysis programs including CLUSTAL V and many of the PHYLIP 3.4 programs. GDE 2.0 is available free of charge for anonymous FTP transfer either at golgi. harvard.edu in directory pub/GDE2.0 or at ftp.bio.indiana.edu in directory molbio/unix/ GDE.

Acknowledgements

I am grateful to Dr E. C. Holmes for comments on the manuscript, and to Dr J. Felsenstein for information on program packages.

References

1. Buonagurio, D. A. *et al.* (1986). *Science*, **232**, 980.
2. Both, G. W. *et al.* (1983). *J. Virol.*, **48**, 52.
3. Daniels, R. S. *et al.* (1985). *J. Gen. Virol.*, **66**, 457.
4. Hayashida, H. *et al.* (1985). *Mol. Biol. Evol.*, **2**, 289.
5. Yamashita, M. *et al.* (1988). *Virology*, **163**, 112.
6. Cox, N. J. *et al.* (1989). *J. Gen. Virol.*, **70**, 299.
7. Donis, R. O. *et al.* (1989). *Virology*, **169**, 408.
8. Alizon, M. *et al.* (1986). *Cell*, **46**, 63.
9. Li, W.-H. *et al.* (1988). *Mol. Biol. Evol.*, **5**, 313.
10. Yokoyama, S. *et al.* (1988). *Mol. Biol. Evol.*, **5**, 237.
11. Smith, T. F. *et al.* (1988). *Nature*, **333**, 573.
12. Balfe, P. *et al.* (1990). *J. Virol.*, **64**, 6221.
13. Myers, G. *et al.* (1992). *Human retroviruses and AIDS 1992*. Los Alamos National Laboratory.

14. Holmes, E. C. *et al.* (1992). *Proc. Natl. Acad. Sci. USA*, **89**, 4835.
15. Chan, S.-Y., *et al.* (1992). *J. Virol.*, **66**, 5714.
16. Rigby, M., *et al.* (1993). *J. Gen. Virol.*, **74**, 425.
17. Simmonds, P., *et al.* (1993). *J. Gen. Virol.*, **74**, 661.
18. Fitch, W. M. (1977). *Amer. Nat.*, **111**, 223.
19. Sokal, R. R. and Sneath, P. H. A. (1963). *Principles of numerical taxonomy.* W. H. Freeman, San Francisco.
20. Nei, M. and Li, W.-H. (1979). *Proc. Natl. Acad. Sci. USA*, **78**, 5269.
21. Jukes, T. H. and Cantor, C. R. (1969). In *Mammalian protein metabolism III* (ed H. N. Munro). Academic Press, New York.
22. Kimura, M. (1980). *J. Mol. Evol.*, **16**, 111
23. Gojobori, T. *et al* (1990). In *Methods in enzymology*, Vol. 183, pp. 531–50.
24. Leigh Brown, A. and Monaghan, P. (1988). *AIDS Res. Hum. Retrovir.*, **4**, 313.
25. Sakaguchi, T. *et al.* (1989). *Virology*, **169**, 260
26. Fitch, W. and Margoliash, E. (1967). *Science*, **155**, 279.
27. Saitou, N. and Nei, M. (1987). *Mol. Biol. Evol.*, **4**, 406.
28. Li, W. H. and Graur, D. (1991). *Fundamentals of molecular evolution.* Sinauer, Sunderland MA.
29. Felsenstein, J. (1988). *Ann. Rev. Genet.*, **22**, 521.
30. Dermody, T. S. *et al.* (1990). *J. Virol.*, **64**, 4842.
31. Felsenstein, J. (1978). *Syst. Zool.*, **27**, 401.
32. Wolfs, T. F. W. *et al.* (1991). *Virology*, **185**, 195.
33. Wolfs, T. F. W. *et al.* (1992). *Virology*, **189**, 103.
34. Felsentein, J. (1985). *Evolution*, **39**, 783.
35. Felsenstein, J. (1981). *J. Mol. Evol.*, **17**, 368.
36. Bishop, M. J. and Friday, A. E. (1985). *Proc. Roy. Soc. Lond. Ser. B.*, **226**, 271.
37. Higgins, D. G. and Sharp, P. M. (1988). *Gene*, **73**, 237.

A1

Addresses of suppliers

Amersham International Plc, Amersham Place, Little Chalfont, Buckingham-shire, HP7 9NA, UK; and 2636 South Clearbrook Drive, Arlington Heights, Illinois, 60005, USA.

Anderman & Co Ltd (for Schleicher & Schuell), 145 London Road, Kingston-upon-Thames, Surrey, KT2 6NH, UK.

Applied Biosystems, Birchwood Science Park North, Warrington, Cheshire, WA3 7PB, UK.

F. Baker Scientific, 6–7 Dalton Court, Astmoor Industrial Estate, Runcorn, Cheshire, WA7 1PU, UK.

BDH Laboratoray Supplies, see Merck Ltd.

Beckman-RIIC Ltd, Progress Road, Sands Industrial Estate, High Wycombe, Bucks, HP12 4JL, UK.

Becton Dickinson (UK) Ltd, Between Town Road, Cowley, Oxford, OX4 3IY, UK.

Bibby Sterilin Ltd, Tiling Drive, Stone, Staffs, ST15 0SA, UK.

Bio101 Inc, P.O. Box 2284, La Jolla, California, 92038–2284, USA; see also *Stratech Scientific Ltd.*

Bioline, Rowlandson House, 289/293 Ballards Lane, Finchley, London, N12 8NP, UK.

Bio-Nuclear Services Ltd, Highland Comfort, Union Hill, Stratton, Bude, Cornwall, EX23 9BL, UK.

Bio-Rad Laboratories Ltd, Bio-Rad House, Maylands Avenue, Hemel Hempstead, Herts, HP2 7TD, UK.

Boehringer Mannheim, Bell Lane, Lewes, East Sussex, BN17 1LG, UK; and P.O. Box 50414, Indianapolis, Indiana, 46250, USA.

Cetus see Perkin Elmer Ltd.

Dako Ltd, 16 Manor Courtyard, Hughenden Avenue, High Wycombe, Bucks, HP13 5RE, UK.

Du Pont (UK) Ltd, Wedgwood Way, Stevenage, Herts SG1 4QN, UK.

Dynal (UK) Ltd, Station House, 26 Grove Street, New Ferry, Wirral, Merseyside, L62 5AZ, UK.

Flow Laboratories Ltd, Woodcock Hill, Harefield Road, Rickmansworth, Herts, WD3 1PQ, UK.

Fluka Chemicals Ltd (Aldrich), The Old Brickyard, New Road, Gillingham, Dorset, SP8 4JL, UK.

General Diagnostics, William R. Warner & Co. Ltd, Unit 59C, Milton Trading Estate, Milton, Abingdon, Oxon, OX14 4RX, UK.

Gilder Grids, Withambrook Industrial Park, Londonthorpe Road, Grantham, Lincolnshire, NG31 9ST, UK.

C.A. Hendley (Essex) Ltd, Oakwood Hill Industrial Estate, Loughton, Essex, UK.

Hoefer Scientific Instruments (UK), Unit 12, Croft Road Workshops, Croft Road, off Hempstalls Lane, Newcastle-under-Lyme, Staffs, ST5 0TW, UK.

Hybaid Ltd (Qiagen), 111–113 Waldegrave Road, Teddington, Middlesex, TW11 7LL, UK.

Jencons (Scientific) Ltd, Cherrycourt Way Industrial Estate, Stanbridge Road, Leighton Buzzard, LU7 8UA, UK.

Kemble Instrument Co Ltd, Marchants Way, Burgess Hill, West Sussex, RH15 8QY, UK.

Life Technologies, P.O. Box 35, Trident House, Renfrew Road, Paisley, PA3 4EF, UK.

Merck Ltd, Merck House, Poole, Dorset, BH15 1TD, UK; and Hunter Boulevard, Magna Park, Lutterworth, Leics, LE17 4XN, UK.

Millipore (UK) Ltd, 11–15 Peterborough Road, Harrow, Middlesex, HA1 2YH, UK; and The Boulevard, Blackmore Lane, Watford, Herts, WD1 8YW, UK.

New England Biolabs, 67 Knowl Piece, Wilbury Way, Hitchin, Herts, SG4 0TY, UK; and CP Laboratories, P.O. Box 22, Bishop's Stortford, Herts, CM33 3DX, UK.

Northumbria Biologicals, Nelson Industrial Estate, Cramlington, Northumberland, NE23 9BL, UK.

Novabiochem (UK) Ltd, Boulevard Industrial Park, Padge Road, Beeston, Nottingham, NG9 2JR, UK.

Nuclear Enterprises, NE Technology, Bath Road, Beenham, Reading, UK.

Oswel DNA Service, Department of Chemistry, University of Edinburgh, West Mains Road, Edinburgh, EH9 3JJ, UK.

Oxoid, Unipath Ltd, Wade Road, Basingstoke, RG24 0PN, UK.

Perkin Elmer Ltd, Post Office Lane, Beaconsfield, Bucks, HP9 1QA, UK; and 761 Main Avenue, Norwalk, Connecticut, 06859, USA.

Pierce Chemical Co., 3747 N. Meridian Road, P.O. Box 117, Rockford, Illinois, 61105, USA.

Pharmacia Ltd, Pharmacia House, Midsummer Boulevard, Milton Keynes, Bucks, MK9 3HP, UK.

Pharmacia Biotech Ltd, 23 Grosvenor Road, St. Albans, Herts, AL1 3AW, UK; and Davy Avenue, Knowlhill, Milton Keynes, MK5 8PH, UK.

Pharmacia LKB Inc, 800 Centennial Avenue, Piscataway, New Jersey, 08854, USA.

Promega, Delta House, Enterprise Road, Chilworth Research Centre, Southampton, Hants, SO1 7NS, UK; and 2800 S. Fish Hatchery Road, Madison, Wisconsin, 53711, USA.

Qiagen, see **Hybaid Ltd.**

Rathburn Chemicals, Crabston Road, Walkerburn, Peebles, UK.

Sarstedt Ltd, 68 Boston Road, Beaumont Leys, Leicester, LE4 1AW, UK.

Sigma Chemical Co, Fancy Road, Poole, Dorset, BH17 7BR, UK; and P.O. Box 14509, St. Louis, Missouri, 63178, USA.

Skatron Instruments Ltd, Unit 11, Studlands Park Avenue, Newmarket, Suffolk, CB8 7DB, UK.

Stratagene, 140 Cambridge Innovation Centre, Cambridge Science Park, Milton Road, Cambridge, CB4 4GF, UK.

Stratech Scientific Ltd (Bio-101), 61–63 Dudley Street, Luton, Beds, LU2 0NP, UK.

Techne, Duxford, Cambridge, CD2 4PZ, UK; and 3700 Brunswick Pike, Princeton, New Jersey, 08540–6192, USA.

Whatman International Ltd, St. Leonard's Road, 20/20 Maidstone, Kent, ME16 0LS, UK.

Index